Blueprints **for your pocket!**

In an effort to answer a need for high yield review books for the elective rotations, Blackwell Publishing now brings you Blueprints in pocket size.

These new Blueprints provide the essential content needed during the shorter rotations. They will also provide the basic content needed for USMLE Steps 2 and 3, or if you were unable to fit in the rotation, these new pocket-sized Blueprints are just what you need.

Each book will focus on the high yield essential content for the most commonly encountered problems of the specialty. Each book features these special appendices:

- Career and residency opportunities
- Commonly prescribed medications
- Self-test Q&A section

Ask for these at your medical bookstore or check them out online at www.blackwellmedstudent.com

Blueprints Anesthesiology
Blueprints Dermatology
Blueprints Gastroenterology
Blueprints Hematology and Oncology
Blueprints Infectious Diseases
Blueprints Pediatric ICU
Blueprints Pediatric Infectious Diseases
Blueprints Ophthalmology
Blueprints Orthopedics
Blueprints Plastic Surgery
Blueprints Urology

BLUEPRINTS
Infectious
Diseases

Samir S. Shah, MD
Attending Physician
Divisions of Infectious Diseases and General Pediatrics
The Children's Hospital of Philadelphia
Assistant Professor
Department of Pediatrics
University of Pennsylvania School of Medicine
Philadelphia, Pennsylvania

Kent K. Hu, MD, MPH
Affiliate Instructor
Department of Medicine
University of Washington
Seattle, Washington

Heidi M. Crane, MD, MPH
Acting Instructor
Division of Allergy and Infectious Diseases
University of Washington
Attending Physician
Harborview Medical Center
Madison HIV specialty clinic
Seattle, Washington

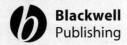

Blackwell
Publishing

Blackwell Publishing, Inc., 350 Main Street,
Malden, Massachusetts 02148-5018, USA
Blackwell Publishing Ltd, 9600 Garsington Road, Oxford OX4 2DQ, UK
Blackwell Publishing Asia Pty Ltd, 550 Swanston Street,
Carlton, Victoria 3053, Australia

05 06 07 08 5 4 3 2 1

ISBN-13: 978-1-4051-0453-1
ISBN-10: 1-4051-0453-8

Library of Congress Cataloging-in-Publication Data

Blueprints infectious diseases/[edited by] Samir S. Shah, Kent K. Hu, Heidi
    M. Crane. p. ; cm.
  Includes index
  ISBN-13: 978-1-4051-0453-1 (pbk. : alk. paper)
  ISBN-10: 1-4051-0453-8 (pbk. : alk. paper) 1. Communicable
    diseases—Handbooks, manuals, etc
  [DNLM: 1. Communicable Diseases—Handbooks. WC 39 B658 2006]
    1. Title Infectious diseases. II. Shah, Samir S. III. Hu, Kent K.
    IV. Crane, Heidi M.

RC112.B68 2006
616.9—dc22

                                                                2005011429

A catalogue record for this title is available from the British Library

Acquisitions: Beverly Copland
Development: Selene Steneck
Production: Debra Murphy
Cover design: Hannus Design Associates
Interior design: Mary McKeon
Typesetter: International Typesetting and Composition in Ft. Lauderdale, FL
Printed and bound by Capital City Press in Berlin, VT

For further information on Blackwell Publishing, visit our website:
www.blackwellmedstudent.com

Notice: The indications and dosages of all drugs in this book have been recommended in the medical literature and conform to the practices of the
general community. The medications described do not necessarily have specific approval by the Food and Drug Administration for use in the diseases
and dosages for which they are recommended. The package insert for each
drug should be consulted for use and dosage as approved by the FDA.
Because standards for usage change, it is advisable to keep abreast of revised
recommendations, particularly those concerning new drugs.

The publisher's policy is to use permanent paper from mills that operate
a sustainable forestry policy, and which has been manufactured from
pulp processed using acid-free and elementary chlorine-free practices.
Furthermore, the publisher ensures that the text paper and cover board used
have met acceptable environmental accreditation standards.

Contents

x • Contents

Contributors

Valerianna Amorosa, MD
Clinical Assistant Professor of Medicine in Infectious Diseases
University of Pennsylvania
Chief of Infectious Diseases
Philadelphia Veterans Affairs Medical Center
Philadelphia, Pennsylvania

Erich Braun, MD
Chief Resident, Ophthalmology
New York University
Manhattan Eye, Ear & Throat Hospital
New York, New York

Corey Casper, MD, MPH
Assistant Professor of Medicine
University of Washington
Assistant Member, Program in Infectious Disease
Fred Hutchinson Cancer Research Center
Associate Medical Director, Infection Control
Seattle Cancer Care Alliance
Seattle, Washington

Maureen Chase, MD
Resident, Emergency Medicine
Hospital of University of Pennsylvania
Jefferson Medical College
Thomas Jefferson University Hospital
Philadelphia, Pennsylvania

Greg Eldon Davis, MD, MPH
Resident, Department of Otolaryngology-Head and Neck Surgery
University of Washington
University of Washington Medical Center
Seattle, Washington

Timothy H. Dellit, MD
Assistant Professor of Medicine
University of Washington School of Medicine
Medical Director, Antimicrobial and Antimicrobial
    Resistance Management
Harborview Medical Center
Seattle, Washington

George A. Diaz, MD
Fellow, Division of Infectious Diseases
Department of Internal Medicine
University of Washington
Seattle, Washington

Erik R. Dubberke, MD
Fellow in Infectious Diseases
Washington University School of Medicine
Barnes-Jewish Hospital
St. Louis, Missouri

Lee S. Engel, MD, PhD
Fellow, Department of Infectious Diseases
Louisiana State University Health Sciences Center
New Orleans, Louisiana

Worth W. Everett, MD
Assistant Professor of Emergency Medicine
University of Pennsylvania
Attending Emergency Physician
Hospital of the University of Pennsylvania
Philadelphia, Pennsylvania

Victoria Fraser, MD
Professor of Medicine
Washington University School of Medicine
Barnes Jewish Hospital
St. Louis, Missouri

Melissa M. Hagman, MD
Acting Instructor of Medicine
University of Washington School of Medicine
University of Washington Medical Center
Seattle, Washington

Peggy Headstrom, MD
Gastroenterology Fellow
University of Washington School of Medicine
Seattle, Washington

Jan V. Hirschmann, MD
Professor, Department of Medicine
University of Washington Medical School
Staff Physician
Puget Sound VA Medical Center
Seattle, Washington

Christopher L. Knight, MD
Assistant Professor of Medicine
University of Washington School of Medicine
Attending Physician
University of Washington Medical Center
Seattle, Washington

Ajit P. Limaye, MD
Assistant Professor, Laboratory Medicine & Medicine
University of Washington
Attending Physician, Infectious Diseases
Co-Director, Clinical Microbiology
University of Washington Medical Center
Seattle, Washington

Brandi M. Limbago, PhD
Senior Microbiology Fellow
Department of Laboratory Medicine
University of Washington
Seattle, Washington

Caroline B. Long, MD
Pediatrics Resident
Children's Hospital of New York at Columbia University
    Medical Center
New York, New York

Fred A. Lopez, MD
Associate Professor and Vice Chair
LSU Department of Medicine
Assistant Dean for Student Affairs
Louisiana State University School of Medicine-New Orleans
New Orleans, Louisiana

Jeanne Marrazzo, MD, MPH
Associate Professor
Department of Medicine, Division of Allergy and Infectious Diseases
University of Washington
Seattle, Washington

Mari Mizuta, MD
Fellow, Division of Infectious Diseases
The Hospital of University of Pennsylvania
Philadelphia, Pennsylvania

Douglas S. Paauw, MD, FACP
Professor of Medicine
University of Washington School of Medicine
Rathman Family Foundation Endowed Chair for Patient-Centered
   Clinical Education
Seattle, Washington

Paul S. Pottinger, MD, DTM&H
Senior Fellow
Department of Medicine
Division of Allergy and Infectious Diseases
University of Washington
Seattle, Washington

Ahmet Tural, MD
Department of Infectious Diseases
Providence Physician Group
Everett, Washington

Theoklis Zaoutis, MD
Assistant Professor, Department of Pediatrics Center for Clinical
   Epidemiology and Biostatistics
University of Pennsylvania Medical School
Director, Antimicrobial Stewardship, Division of Infectious Diseases
The Children's Hospital of Philadelphia
Philadelphia, Pennsylvania

Reviewers

Pamneit Bhogal
4th year student
Temple University School of Medicine
Philadelphia, Pennsylvania

Jojy George, MD
Resident, Department of Surgery
University of Tennessee
Memphis, Tennessee

Amir A. Ghaferi
4th year student
Johns Hopkins University School of Medicine
Baltimore, Maryland

David Gloss, MD, MPH & TM
Resident
Tulane University, Medicine/Neurology
New Orleans, Louisiana

Sandy Green
4th year student
Temple School of Medicine
Philadelphia, Pennsylvania

Padi McFadden
4th year student
University of Pittsburgh School of Medicine
Pittsburgh, Pennsylvania

Anil Nair, MD
Resident, Neurosurgery
Albany Medical Center
Albany, New York

Preface

Blueprints have become the standard for medical students to use during their clerkship rotations and sub-internships and as a review book for taking the USMLE Steps 2 and 3.

Blueprints initially were only available for the five main specialties: medicine, pediatrics, obstetrics and gynecology, surgery, and psychiatry. Students found these books so valuable that they asked for Blueprints in other topics and so family medicine, emergency medicine, neurology, cardiology, and radiology were added.

In an effort to answer a need for high-yield review books for the elective rotations, Blackwell Publishing now brings you Blueprints in pocket size. These books are developed to provide students in the shorter, elective rotations, often taken in 4th year, with the same high-yield, essential contents of the larger Blueprints books. These new pocket-sized Blueprints will be invaluable for those students who need to know the essentials of a clinical area but were unable to take the rotation. Students in physician assistant, nurse practitioner, and osteopath programs will find these books meet their needs for the clinical specialties.

Feedback from student reviewers give high praise for this addition to the Blueprints brand. Each of these new books was developed to be read in a short time period and to address the basics needed during a particular clinical rotation. Please see the Series Page for a list of the books that you can find in your bookstore or on our website at www.blackwellmedstudent.com.

Acknowledgments

We thank our colleagues who have contributed their expertise in writing chapters for this book. We would also like to thank our Department chairs, Drs. Alan Cohen, Walter Stamm, and Bill Bremner for creating an environment supportive of intellectual pursuits. We appreciate the wise counsel and support of our Division Chiefs, Drs. Paul Offit, Louis Bell, King Holmes, and Steve Fihn. Over the years, we have also learned from many other excellent clinicians and mentors such as Drs. Stephen Ludwig, William Schwartz, Joshua Metlay, Mari Kitahata, Bob Harrington, and Sanjay Saint. Their dedication to teaching and research and commitment to patient care are attributes we strive to emulate. We also wish to thank Dr. Paul Crane for his careful reading of the proofs. Finally, we offer thanks to our family, friends, and colleagues who provided encouragements and support for this project.

Abbreviations

3TC	lamivudine
5-FC	flucytosine
A-a	alveolar-arterial
ABC	abacavir
ABC/AZT/3TC	Trizivir
ABR	acute bacterial rhinosinusitis
ACTH	adrenocorticotropic hormone
AFB	acid-fast bacilli
AIDS	acquired immunodeficiency syndrome
ANC	absolute neutrophil count
AOE	acute otitis externa
AOM	acute otitis media
APV	amprenavir
ARDS	acute respiratory distress syndrome
ASA	aspirin
ATV	atazanavir
AZT	zidovudine
AZT/3TC	Combivir
BCG	bacille Calmette-Guérin vaccine
BCYE	buffered charcoal yeast extract
BMT	bilateral myringotomy and tube placement
BRAT	bananas, rice, applesauce, toast
BSI	bloodstream infection
BUN	blood urea nitrogen
BV	bacterial vaginosis
C&S	culture and sensitivity
CAD	coronary artery disease
CAP	community-acquired pneumonia
CBC	complete blood count
CDC	Centers for Disease Control and Prevention
CFU	colony-forming unit
CHF	congestive heart failure
CI	contraindicated
CMV	cytomegalovirus
CNA	colistin naladixic acid
CNS	central nervous system
COM	chronic otitis media
COPD	chronic obstructive pulmonary disease
CQ	chloroquine
CRP	C-reactive protein

CRS	chronic rhinosinusitis
CSF	cerebrospinal fluid
CSOM	chronic suppurative otitis media
CT	chloridic trachonedis
CT	computed tomography
CTF	Colorado tick fever
CVC	central venous catheter
CXR	chest x-ray
CYP-450	cytochrome P-450
d4T	stavudine
ddC	zalcitabine
DDI	didanosine
DFA	direct fluorescent antibody
DIC	disseminated intravascular coagulation
DLV	delavirdine
DOT	directly observed therapy
DVT	deep venous thrombosis
EBNA	Epstein-Barr nuclear antigen
EBV	Epstein-Barr virus
ECG	electrocardiogram
EEG	electroencephalogram
EFV	efavirenz
EGD	esophagogastroduodenoscopy
EHEC	enterohemorrhagic E. coli
EIA	enzyme immunosorbent assay
EIEC	enteroinvasive E. coli
ELISA	enzyme-linked immunosorbent assay
EMB	ethambutol
ENF/T-20	enfuvirtide
EPEC	enteropathogenic E. coli
ERCP	endoscopic retrograde cholangiopancreatography
ESBLs	extended spectrum beta-lactamases
ESR	erythrocyte sedimentation rate
ETEC	enterotoxigenic E. coli
F-APV	fosamprenavir
FMF	familial Mediterranean fever
FTA-ABS	fluorescent treponemal antibody absorption test
FTC	emtricitabine
FUO	fever of unknown origin
GABHS	group A beta-hemolytic streptococcus
GC	Neisseria gonorrhoeae
GCSF	granulocyte colony-stimulating factor
GERD	gastroesophageal reflux disease
GNR	gram-negative rods
gp41	glycoprotein 41
GS	Gram stain
GUD	genital ulcer disease
GVHD	graft-versus-host disease

HA	headache
HAART	highly active antiretroviral therapy
HACEK	*Haemophilus* spp, *Actinobacillus actinomycetemcomitans, Cardiobacterium hominis, Eikenella corrodens,* and *Kingella kingae*
HAV	hepatitis A virus
HBcAb	antibody to hepatitis B core antigen
HBeAb	antibody to hepatitis B envelope antigen
HBeAg	hepatitis B envelope antigen
HBsAb	antibody to hepatitis B surface antigen
HBsAg	hepatitis B surface antigen
HBV	hepatitis B virus
HCV	hepatitis C virus
HCW	healthcare worker
HGE	human granulocytic ehrlichiosis
HHV	human herpes virus
HIB	*Haemophilus influenzae* type B vaccine
HIV	human immunodeficiency virus
HME	human monocytic ehrlichiosis
HPV	human papillomavirus
HSV	herpes simplex virus
HSV-1	herpes simplex virus, type 1
HSV-2	herpes simplex virus, type 2
HTLV	human T cell lymphotropic virus
HUS	hemolytic-uremic syndrome
hyper-IgD	hyperimmunoglobulinemia D
ICU	intensive care unit
IDU	injection drug users
IDV	indinavir
Ig	immunoglobulin
IgG	immunoglobulin G
IgM	immunoglobulin M
IM	intramuscular
INH	isoniazid
IPV	inactivated poliovirus vaccine
IVDA	intravenous drug abuse
IVIG	intravenous immunoglobulin
KOH	potassium hydroxide
KS	Kaposi's sarcoma
LAD	lymphadenopathy
LDH	lactate dehydrogenase
LFT	liver function tests
LP	lumbar puncture
LPV	lopinavir
LRTI	lower respiratory tract infection
MAC	*Mycobacterium avium-intracellulare complex*
MAP	mean arterial pressure
MBC	minimum bactericidal concentration
MCD	multicentric Castleman's disease

MDR	multidrug-resistant
MEFV	Mediterranean fever gene
MI	myocardial infarction
MIC	minimum inhibitory concentration
MODS	multiple organ dysfunction syndrome
MRI	magnetic resonance imaging
MRSA	methicillin-resistant *Staphylococcus aureus*
MSM	men who have sex with men
MSSA	methicillin-sensitive *Staphylococcus aureus*
MTX	methotrexate
MVP	mitral valve prolapse
NCCLS	National Committee for Clinical Laboratory Standards
NFV	nelfinavir
NLD	nasolacrimal duct
NLF	nelfinavir
NNRTI	non-nucleoside reverse transcriptase inhibitors
NRTI	nucleoside reverse transcriptase inhibitor
NSAID	nonsteroidal anti-inflammatory drug
NSI	needle-stick injury
NtRTI	nucleotide reverse transcriptase inhibitor
NVP	nevirapine
O&P	ova and parasite
OCP	oral contraceptive
OI	opportunistic infection
OME	otitis media with effusion
OPV	oral poliovirus vaccine
p-ANCA	perinuclear antineutrophil cytoplasmic antibodies
PaO2	arterial partial pressure of oxygen
PBP	penicillin binding protein
PCN	penicillin
PCP	*Pneumocystis jiroveci* pneumonia (previously known as *Pneumocystis carinii* pneumonia)
PCR	polymerase chain reaction
PDA	patent ductus arteriosus
PEL	primary effusion lymphoma
PEP	postexposure prophylaxis
PI	protease inhibitor
PICC	percutaneous inserted central catheter
PID	pelvic inflammatory disease
PIV	parainfluenza
PMC	pseudomembranous colitis
PMN	polymorphonuclear cell
PO	per os (by mouth)
PPD	purified protein derivative
PT	prothrombin time
PTT	partial thromboplastin time
PTLD	post-transplant lymphoproliferative disease

PZA	pyrazinamide
RA	rheumatoid arthritis
RIF	rifampin
RIF-PZA	rifampin-pyrazinamide
RIG	rabies immunoglobulin
RMSF	Rocky Mountain spotted fever
RPR	rapid plasma reagin
RSV	respiratory syncytial virus
RTV	ritonavir
SARS	severe acute respiratory syndrome
SIADH	syndrome of inappropriate antidiuretic hormone
SLE	systemic lupus erythematosus
SPE	streptococcal pyrogenic exotoxin
SPICE	*Serratia, Pseudomonas, Providencia,* indole-positive *Proteus, Citrobacter, Enterobacter, Morganella*
SQV-HGC	saquinavir hard gel capsule
SQV-SGC	saquinavir soft gel capsule
STD	sexually transmitted disease
TB	tuberculosis
Td	tetanus and diphtheria
TEE	transesophageal echocardiogram
TIG	tetanus immunoglobulin
TM	tympanic membrane
TMP/SMX	trimethoprim-sulfamethoxazole
TNF	tenofovir
TNF-receptor	tumor necrosis factor receptor
TOA	tubo-ovarian abscess
TPPA	*Treponema pallidum* particle agglutination
TRAPS	tumor necrosis factor receptor-associated periodic syndrome
TSS	toxic shock syndrome
TSST-1	toxic shock syndrome toxin-1
TTE	transthoracic echocardiogram
U/A	urinalysis
URI	upper respiratory infection
UTI	urinary tract infection
VA	ventriculoatrial
VATS	video-assisted thoracoscopy
VCA	viral capsid antigen
VDRL	Venereal Disease Research Laboratory
VHF	viral hemorrhagic fever
VIG	vaccinia immunoglobulin
VOD	veno-occlusive disease
VP	ventriculoperitoneal
VRE	vancomycin-resistant *Enterococcus*
VZV	varicella-zoster virus
WBC	white blood cell (count)
WHO	World Health Organization

1 Diagnostic Microbiology

Brandi M. Limbago, PhD and Ajit P. Limaye, MD

Laboratory Methods Used to Identify Bacteria

■ **Direct Examination** (Table 1-1)

- **Microscopic morphology:** Cocci, rods, chains, clusters, spores, etc.
- **Gram stain: Purple, gram-positive; red/pink, gram-negative**
  - Based on cell wall composition
  - Some do not stain or stain unpredictably (*Mycobacterium, Mycoplasma, Nocardia*)
- **Acid-fast stains:** Auramine-rhodamine, Kinyoun, modified Kinyoun, Ziehl-Neelsen
  - Organisms are resistant to decolorization with acid due to mycolic acids in cell wall
  - Used for *Mycobacterium, Nocardia, Rhodococcus,* and others

■ **Growth on Culture Media**

- Macroscopic morphology on culture
  - Colony size, shape, motility, color, and time for growth
  - **Hemolysis** and lactose fermentation
- Atmospheric requirements
  - Aerobic, microaerophilic, anaerobic, capnophilic
- Blood agar: Supports growth of many common bacteria
  - **Not** *Haemophilus, Neisseria,* other fastidious organisms
  - Can determine hemolysis
- **Chocolate agar: *Haemophilus, Neisseria***
- MacConkey and eosin-methylene blue
  - Useful for gastrointestinal organisms
  - **Differentiate lactose fermenters** (*Eschericia coli, Klebsiella, Enterobacter*) from non-lactose fermenters (*Salmonella, Shigella, Pseudomonas, Acinetobacter*)
- Specialized culture media
  - Supplemented to enrich for organisms that do not grow on routine media (e.g., buffered charcoal yeast extract [BCYE] agar, Brucella agar)
  - Contains compounds that inhibit faster-growing microflora (e.g., selenite broth, colistin nalidixic acid [CNA] agar)

■ TABLE 1-1 General Classification of Organisms Encountered in the Clinical Microbiology Laboratory

Gram-positive cocci

Aerobic	Enterococcus, Micrococcus, Pediococcus, Staphylococcus, Streptococcus
Anaerobic	Anaerococcus, Peptococcus, Peptostreptococcus

Gram-positive bacilli
Aerobic

Spore-forming	Bacillus, Brevibacillus, Paenibacillus
Non-spore forming	Erysipelothrix, Listeria, Corynebacterium, Gardnerella, Gordonia, Rhodococcus, Rothia
Branching	Nocardia, Streptomyces, Tsukamurella

Anaerobic

Spore-forming	Clostridium
Non-spore forming	Bifidobacterium, Eubacterium, Lactobacillus, Mobiluncus, Propionibacterium
Branching	Actinomyces

Gram-negative cocci

Aerobic	Moraxella, Neisseria
Anaerobic	Veillonella, Acidaminococcus, Megasphaera

Gram-negative bacilli
Aerobic

Coliform	Citrobacter, Edwardsiella, Enterobacter, Escherichia, Hafnia, Klebsiella, Morganella, Proteus, Providencia, Salmonella, Shigella, Serratia, Yersinia
Noncoliform	Acinetobacter, Aeromonas, Burkholderia, Plesiomonas, Pseudomonas, Stenotrophomonas
Curved or spiral	Campylobacter, Helicobacter, Leptospira, Vibrio
Fastidious	Afipia, Bartonella, Bordetella, Brucella, Francisella, Haemophilus, Legionella, Pasteurella
Other	Achromobacter, Alcaligenes, Chryseobacterium, Methylobacterium, Oligella, Ralstonia, Roseomonas, Shewanella, Sphingomonas, Weeksella

Anaerobic

Bacilli	Bacteroides, Bilophila, Desulfovibrio, Fusobacterium, Leptotrichia, Porphyromonas, Prevotella
Spirochetes	Borrelia, Brachyspira, Spirillum, Treponema mucogenicum

Bacteria that do not Gram stain	Anaplasma, Bartonella, Chlamydia, Coxiella, Erlichia, Mycoplasma, Rickettsia, Ureaplasma

■ TABLE 1-1   Continued

Acid fast Slow-growing	*Mycobacterium tuberculosis, M. avium-intracellulare* complex (MAC), *M. bovis, M. hemophilum, M. kansasii, M. leprae, M. marinum, M. smegmatis, M. ulcerans, M. xenopi*
Fast-growing	*M. abscessus, M. chelonae, M. fortuitum, M. mucogenicum*
Fungi Yeasts	*Candida, Cryptococcus, Malassezia, Pneumocystis, Rhodotorula, Saccharomyces, Trichosporon*
Molds	*Acremonium, Alternaria, Aspergillus, Bipolaris, Cladophialophora,* Dermatophytes (e.g., *Epidermophyton, Microsporum, Trichophyton,* etc.) *Exophiala, Fusarium, Microsporum, Paecilomyces, Penicillium, Scedosporium,* Zygomycetes (e.g., *Mucor, Rhizopus*)
Dimorphic	*Blastomyces, Coccidioides, Histoplasma, Paracoccidioides, Sporothrix*
Parasites Protozoa	*Acanthamoeba* spp, *Babesia microti, Balamuthia mandrillaris, Cryptosporidium parvum, Cyclospora cayetanensis, Dientamoeba fragilis, Encephalitozoon* spp, *Enterocytozoon* spp, *Entamoeba* spp, *Giardia lamblia, Isospora belli, Leishmania* spp, *Plasmodium* spp, *Sarcocystis* spp, *Toxoplasma gondii, Trichomonas vaginalis, Trypanosoma* spp
Trematodes (flukes)	*Clonorchis sinensis, Fasciola* spp, *Gastrodiscoides hominis, Opisthorchis* spp, *Paragonimus* spp, *Schistosoma* spp
Cestodes (tapeworms)	*Diphyllobothrium* spp, *Echinococcus* spp, *Hymenolepsis* spp, *Spirometra* spp, *Taenia* spp
Nematodes (roundworms)	*Ancyclostoma* spp, *Ascaris lumbricoides, Brugia malayi, Dracunculus medinensis, Enterobius vermicularis, Necator americanus, Onchocerca volvulus, Strongyloides* spp, *Trichinella spiralis, Trichuris trichiura, Wuchereria bancrofti*

■ **Direct Specimen Diagnostic Testing**
- Detection of antigens, DNA, or antibodies
- Useful for organisms that are nonculturable, fastidious, slow-growing
  - Urine antigen test to detect *Legionella pneumophila* serogroup 1
  - Toxin A and B detection for *Clostridium difficile*

■ Commercial Systems

- Based on substrate utilization, enzyme production, carbohydrate fermentation, or biochemical reactions converted to a code and compared with database

Laboratory Methods Used to Identify Fungi

■ Classification (see Table 1-1)

- **Yeasts:** Single-celled, round or oval
- **Moulds:** Multicellular, can have hyphal structures, produce spores; some are dimorphic (can be yeast or mold)

■ Direct Examination

- **Staining characteristics:** Several commonly used fungal stains
  - Calcofluor white: Fluorochrome binds cellulose and chitin
  - Fluorescin-conjugated antibodies or probes detect antigens or DNA
  - Gomori methenamine silver: Pathology stain for tissue
  - Potassium hydroxide: Nails, skin, hair
  - **India ink:** Shows presence of yeast capsule (*Cryptococcus neoformans*)
  - Wright-Giemsa: Useful for bone marrow, blood smears
- **Microscopic morphology**
  - **Yeasts:** Round vs. oval, broad-based vs. narrow-based budding, capsule
  - **Moulds:** Septate vs. nonseptate hyphae, angle of branching

■ Detection of Antigen, Metabolite, or Antibody

- Capsular polysaccharide antigen test for *C. neoformans*

Laboratory Methods Used to Identify Parasites

Most parasites are identified by macroscopic and microscopic morphology, occasionally by antigen or antibody detection (see Table 1-1).

■ Direct Examination

- **Staining characteristics**
  - Auramine-rhodamine: Used for *Cryptosporidium, Isospora*
  - Iron hematoxylin: Detection of protozoan cysts and trophozoites
  - Modified acid-fast: Used for *Cryptosporidium, Isospora, Cyclospora*
  - Wheatley trichrome: Detection of protozoan cysts and trophozoites
  - Wright-Giemsa: Detection of blood parasites

- **Ova and parasite (O&P) exam** (three parts): Requires specimens collected on three consecutive days
  - Direct exam with wet mount for worms, larvae, and motility
  - Concentrated exam for ova, cysts, and larvae
  - Stained exam for intestinal protozoan cysts and trophozoites

Antibiotic Susceptibility Testing

- Used to predict clinical outcome based on an organism's *in vitro* susceptibility to antibiotics
- Many host- and organism-specific factors crucial to clinical outcome cannot be assessed in the laboratory
- In general, *in vitro* resistance is a better predictor of clinical failure than susceptibility is of success
- Clinical isolates are cultured in the presence of antimicrobial agents to determine the concentration of antibiotic required to inhibit growth
- Results for each organism-drug combination are reported as **susceptible (S), intermediate (I),** or **resistant (R)** [according to Clinical and Laboratory Standards Institute (CLSI), formerly National Committee for Clinical Laboratory Standards (NCCLS) breakpoints (Table 1-2)]

■ Important Terms

- **Minimum inhibitory concentration (MIC):** Lowest concentration of a given agent required to **inhibit growth** of an organism
- **Minimum bactericidal concentration (MBC):** Lowest concentration of a given agent required to **kill 99.9%** of the original inoculum
- **Breakpoints:** Interpretive thresholds established by the CLSI for defining susceptibility of clinical isolates. Criteria are determined by microbiological, pharmacological, clinical, and research considerations, and are organism-drug specific. CLSI interpretive criteria do not exist for all organism-drug combinations

■ Methods of Antibiotic Susceptibility Testing

Broth Methods

- **Macrodilution:** Test tubes containing serial dilutions of an antibiotic in a broth medium are inoculated with a standardized suspension of organism and incubated under standardized conditions. The first concentration at which no growth is detected is defined as the MIC for that organism to that drug. MBC is determined by plating an aliquot from concentrations at and above the MIC onto solid media. The first concentration

■ TABLE 1-2   Antibiotic Susceptibility Testing

		CLSI Standardized Method	CLSI Breakpoints Available	Adaptable*	Time (Hours)	Ease of Performance	Cost
Dilution	Broth microdilution	Yes	Yes	Yes	16–24	Moderate	$
	Broth dilution MIC	Yes	Yes	Yes	16–24	Moderate	$
	Broth dilution MBC	Yes	Yes	Yes	40–48	Difficult	$$
	Agar dilution	Yes	Yes	Yes	16–24	Difficult	$
Diffusion	Disk diffusion	Yes	Yes	No	16–24	Easy	$
	E-test	Yes	Yes	Yes	16–24	Easy	$
Specialized	Schlichter	Yes	No	No	16–24	Moderate	$$
	Synergy testing	Yes	No	No	16–24	Difficult	$$$

* Method can be adapted for testing of fastidious organisms.

to demonstrate **99.9% fewer colonies than the original inoculum** is defined as the MBC for that organism-drug combination

- **Microdilution:** Similar to macrodilution, except that the assay is performed with smaller volumes of broth in a microtiter plate rather than in test tubes
- **Automated testing systems:** Some instruments have the capacity to perform a version of the broth microdilution technique on a real-time basis. Bacterial suspensions in the presence of increasing antibiotic concentrations are incubated and monitored optically at regular intervals (usually 15–30 minutes), allowing for a more rapid determination of MIC

Agar Methods

- **Agar dilution:** Agar plates containing defined concentrations of each antibiotic to be tested are prepared and inoculated with a standardized suspension of the test organism. Plates are then incubated aerobically for 16–24 hours and examined for growth. The lowest concentration of antibiotic to inhibit visible growth is recorded as the MIC
- **Agar diffusion**
  - **Kirby-Bauer disk diffusion:** A standardized suspension of organism is plated for confluent growth on solid media, and paper disks impregnated with an antibiotic are placed onto the agar. During overnight incubation, each drug diffuses into the agar, producing a circular concentration gradient of antibiotic around the disk. The diameter of the zone of growth inhibition around each antibiotic disk correlates well with MIC values, allowing classification of the organism as S, I, or R based on the zone diameter
  - **Gradient diffusion (E test):** A standardized bacterial suspension is plated for confluent growth on an agar medium, and a plastic strip impregnated with a gradient of antibiotic is placed onto the agar. During overnight incubation, drug diffuses into the agar, producing an ellipsoidal concentration gradient of antibiotic surrounding the strip and, consequently, an ellipsoidal zone of growth inhibition. The base of the ellipse is measured against values delineated on the strip to obtain an MIC for that organism

Molecular Testing

The presence of a particular gene or mutation is often associated with an established resistance profile in specific organisms (e.g., *mecA* and methicillin resistance in staphylococci). In these cases, the genotype, rather than the associated phenotype, can be assayed directly. This approach is very sensitive and does not necessarily require culture of the test organism, but is limited by the relatively high cost of molecular testing and lack of well-characterized genetic determinants associated with resistance in some organisms

Specialized Testing

- **Synergy testing:** A combination of two drugs often has different antibiotic activity than can be accounted for by each of the compounds individually
  - **Synergy** occurs when combinations of two (or more) compounds result in enhanced killing or growth inhibition
  - **Antagonism** occurs when killing or growth inhibition is suppressed by the combination
  - Performed by the checkerboard method, a modification of microbroth dilution, in which one antibiotic is titrated against the other
  - Relatively expensive and labor-intensive, and is therefore **used selectively** in certain clinical situations (e.g., endocarditis, severely immunocompromised patients, life-threatening infections)
- **Schlichter test:** Test of serum bactericidal activity (**not commonly used**)
  - Serial dilutions of the patient's serum are inoculated with the patient's infecting isolate, and both MIC and MBC assays are performed
  - The lowest dilution of the patient's serum to show growth inhibition is interpreted as the fold-coverage in the serum (e.g., a 1:4 dilution implies that the inhibitory concentration in serum is four times that of the MIC)
  - The clinical utility of the Schlichter test is debated, although it may be **useful to monitor therapy for endocarditis and osteomyelitis**

See **Appendix D** for a **summary** of clinical syndromes, causative organisms, and preferred diagnostic tests.

Clinical and Diagnostic Virology

Corey Casper, MD, MPH

Typical Virus Classification

- (1) Nucleic acid structure: DNA vs. RNA and single stranded vs. double stranded; (2) presence or absence of envelope; (3) organization of genome, mode of transcription
- May be more useful to classify by clinical manifestations
  - Those causing similar syndromes (respiratory viruses, gastrointestinal viruses, hemorrhagic viruses, etc.)
  - Those with similar treatments (e.g., herpesviruses)

Diagnosis

- Direct
  - Viral culture: May detect many viruses, gives antiviral susceptibilities, but may take ≥72 hours, and is insensitive
  - Polymerase chain reaction (PCR): Exponential amplification of small amounts of nucleic acids for rapid diagnosis and **high sensitivity,** but poorer specificity due to contamination or detection of virus unrelated to acute illness
  - Direct fluorescent antibody (DFA): Detects viral antigens in clinical specimens. **Rapid, specific, but lacks sensitivity** of PCR and susceptibility information from culture
- Indirect: Serum antibodies to viral proteins. Detection of IgM, indicating early infection, is often technically challenging and prone to **poor specificity.** Detection of IgG not typically useful in management of acute illness

HUMAN HERPESVIRUSES (HHV)

■ Characteristics

- Eight types of HHV, worldwide distribution, very prevalent
- Large viruses with double-stranded DNA and lipid envelope
- Lifelong infection. Life cycle varies between latent ("hibernating") and lytic (active viral replication, often associated with symptoms) phases
- Severe sequelae in persons with impaired cellular immunity

Herpes Simplex Virus, Type 1 (HSV-1)

- **50% to 90% of people infected worldwide**
- Most infections occur in childhood via saliva, leading to **life-long latency in nerve ganglia** (usually trigeminal)
- Typically cause episodic "cold sores" or "fever blisters," but increasingly recognized as cause of genital herpes. May also cause encephalitis, pneumonitis, and hepatitis
- Diagnosis: (1) Direct: Culture, DFA, or PCR of lesion by unroofing lesion and scraping base; (2) Indirect: *Type-specific* antibody test (ELISA or Western Blot)
- Treatment: Oral or intravenous acyclovir, valacyclovir, famciclovir (topical preparations rarely effective). Treat resistant virus (rare in absence of HIV) with IV foscarnet

Herpes Simplex Virus, Type 2 (HSV-2)
(see also Chapter 12)

- 25% of people in the US infected, but largely underdiagnosed
- Most infections occur during adolescence/young adulthood, through direct contact between mucosal surfaces
- After primary infection, virus travels to sacral ganglia. May recur at skin surface in the sacral dermatomal distribution
- Virus is shed on days when infected person has no symptoms, accounting for majority of transmissions
- Episodes start with a prodrome of **local pain/dysesthesias** (constitutional symptoms common with primary infection) for 4 to 6 days. Progress to vesicular lesion over 1 to 2 weeks, followed by ulceration and crusting by 3 weeks
- Less common complications: Encephalitis (especially among neonates) and hepatitis
- Diagnosis and treatment: As with HSV-1

Varicella-Zoster Virus (VZV)

- 90% of adults have antibodies to VZV
- Primary infection causes chickenpox, followed by latency in dorsal ganglia of spinal cord. Subsequent reactivation in dorsal nerve ganglia leads to herpes zoster ("shingles"), a vesicular rash in dermatomal distribution
- May also cause pneumonitis, hepatitis, retinal necrosis
- Treatment with acyclovir, valacyclovir, or famciclovir in disseminated primary infection, the immunocompromised host, or herpes zoster
- Diagnosis: (1) Direct: **DFA** from unroofing lesion and scraping base; (2) Indirect: Serum antibody test (ELISA)

Epstein-Barr Virus (EBV)

- 90% infected with virus, most before adulthood, through contact with saliva
- Primary infection causes mononucleosis (pharyngitis, fever, lymphadenopathy, splenomegaly)
- Latency in B cells may lead to malignancy in future: Hodgkin's disease, Burkitt's lymphoma, posttransplantation lymphoproliferative disease
- Diagnosis: **Monospot** as first test, but **may miss 30% of cases and incorrectly diagnose 10%** of people without mono. EBV serologies: EBV viral capsid antigen (VCA) IgM + with Epstein-Bair nuclear antigen (EBNA) IgG—suggests acute EBV infection
- Antivirals not used (except in hemophagocytic syndrome)

Cytomegalovirus (CMV)

- 70% of people in US infected by adulthood. Virus frequently secreted in saliva/urine of asymptomatic persons
- Primary infection mimics mononucleosis
- Reactivation in immunocompromised host leads to retinitis (HIV), colitis (HIV or transplant), pneumonitis (transplant), hepatitis, fever of unknown origin
- Diagnosis: Viral culture or PCR
- Treatment: Ganciclovir or foscarnet are drugs of choice

HHV-6/7

- Over 95% of people in US have serum antibodies to HHV-6
- Causes roseola infantum and fevers, usually 6 to 12 months old
- Meningitis in organ transplant patients and pneumonitis in AIDS patients
- Diagnosis: PCR
- Treatment: IV ganciclovir may be effective

HHV-8 (Kaposi's Sarcoma-Associated Herpesvirus)

- Up to 5% of US population has serum antibodies, but higher among men who have sex with men (25% to 50%), persons from Southern Mediterranean or Middle East (30%), and Africa (30% to 100%)
- Causes Kaposi's sarcoma (KS), primary effusion lymphoma (PEL) and multicentric Castleman's disease (MCD)
- Diagnosis: PCR or serology by ELISA
- Treatment: Antiretroviral therapy for AIDS-associated KS; chemotherapy for KS, PEL, and MCD

RESPIRATORY VIRUSES

- Seasonal
  - Influenza and SARS: Late fall/early winter
  - Coronaviruses (including SARS): Winter
  - Respiratory syncytial virus (RSV) and metapneumovirus: Winter/spring
  - Adenovirus: Year-round
  - Parainfluenza (PIV): Fall (PIV-1 and 2) or spring (PIV-3)
  - Rhinovirus: Fall and spring
- Transmitted from respiratory droplets to upper respiratory tract or conjunctiva
- Severe sequelae in the immunocompromised

Influenza

- Two types: A (rapidly mutates via antigenic drift) and B (stable)
- Typically presents as fever, myalgias, cough, rhinitis
- Complications: Bacterial superinfection in lungs (usually pneumococcus or *Staphylococcus aureus*), hepatitis, myositis, Guillain-Barré, and encephalitis
- Diagnosis: **DFA** or culture, **PCR** becoming more common
- Treatment: (1) Vaccine effective against types A and B; (2) amantadine and rimantadine for type A only, also prophylaxis for high risk unvaccinated persons; (3) neuraminidase inhibitors oseltamivir (oral) and zanamivir (inhaled) are effective against types A and B

Respiratory Syncytial Virus

- Usually presents as upper respiratory infection (URI), usually acquired by age 3. Can progress to lower tract infection (LRTI) (especially in transplant patients) manifesting as bronchospasm and pneumonia
- Diagnosis: **DFA,** culture, or PCR
- Treatment: Supportive, although inhaled ribavirin may be useful in some children and adult transplant patients

Adenovirus

- Common cause of URI and keratoconjuntivitis. Has been occasionally associated with pneumonia in community outbreaks, diarrhea in children, and hepatitis
- May cause cystitis or nephritis in transplant patients

- Diagnosis: **PCR**, culture, and DFA
- Treatment: Supportive; IV cidofovir in immunocompromised

Parainfluenza

- Common cause of URI. In children, leading cause of croup. Can cause severe LRTI in some children/transplant patients
- Diagnosis: Culture, **DFA,** PCR
- Treatment: Supportive

Rhinovirus

- Leading cause of the "common cold." Transmitted by nasal secretions to nasal/conjunctival mucosa
- URI symptoms persist for 1 to 2 weeks, and may be complicated by bacterial otitis or sinusitis
- Diagnosis: Culture, PCR
- Treatment: Supportive

Metapneumovirus

- Recently identified from retrospective series of unidentified respiratory illnesses
- Serologic studies suggest most are infected by 5 years of age, peak 6 to 12 months
- Mild URI in most, with rare progression to severe LRTI
- Diagnosis: PCR
- Treatment: Not established

Coronaviruses

- Large family of viruses with multiple animal hosts
- Usually nonspecific symptoms such as fevers, myalgias, fatigue. May progress to nonproductive cough and dyspnea
- Diagnosis: PCR
- Treatment: Supportive

SARS

- Newly identified virus associated with severe LRTI in Asia and elsewhere in 2003
- Thought to be transmitted by contact with small mammals (civets) in Asia, spread between humans via respiratory droplets and feces
- Respiratory failure develops in minority

GASTROINTESTINAL VIRUSES

- Most common viruses to cause gastrointestinal illnesses are noroviruses, caliciviruses, rotaviruses, astroviruses, and adenoviruses
- Present with diarrhea, fever, and/or abdominal pain. Children more often affected, although incidence high in institutional or "closed" settings (e.g., cruise ships)
- Transmission via fecal-oral route
- Diagnosis: **Antigen detection** or PCR
- Treatment: Supportive

ENTEROVIRUSES

- Large group of viruses including the subgroups polioviruses, echoviruses, and coxsackieviruses
- Worldwide pathogens with most infections in summer and fall

Poliovirus

- Polio has been targeted for worldwide eradication, but recently causes of polio have been documented in areas where vaccination coverage is incomplete. A very small number of annual cases may also be attributed to the live viral vaccine.
- Infection via **fecal-oral transmission**
- Range of symptoms, from asymptomatic infection to paralysis. **Meningitis** is common. Paralytic cases (<1% of infections) start with myalgias, followed by dysesthesias, spasm, and flaccid paralysis *without sensory loss*

Echovirus/Coxsackievirus/ Other Enteroviruses

- Common causes of aseptic meningitis
- Heterogeneous and nondistinct exanthems (skin rashes). Exception: Hand-foot-mouth (coxsackievirus A16) with oral vesicles and papules/vesicles on palms and soles
- Complications: Group A coxsackieviruses may cause herpangina (dysphagia with lesions on soft palate); group B coxsackieviruses can lead to myopericarditis and acute hemorrhagic conjunctivitis with enterovirus 70; and all may cause chronic meningoencephalitis among persons with agammaglobulinemia
- Diagnosis: PCR
- Treatment: Supportive

POXVIRUSES AND PAPILLOMAVIRUSES

Smallpox (Variola), Other Orthopox, and Parapox Viruses

- Smallpox is the only infectious disease eradicated with vaccination, now threatening to return due to bioterrorism
- Infection via respiratory droplets or contact with infected lesions. Acquisition largely asymptomatic for first 7 to 10 days, followed by a nonspecific prodrome: Fevers and malaise
- Patient becomes infectious upon development of rash. Rash typically maculopapular, starts in the oropharynx, head/neck, upper extremities, and moves caudally. Lesions usually *in the same stage* (i.e., vesicular, pustular, crusted), which differentiates the lesion from varicella
- Diagnosis: PCR or electron microscopy of vesicular fluid
- Treatment: Supportive, although **cidofovir** may be effective if given early after infection. **Vaccination within 4 days of exposure may mitigate course of infection**
- **Other orthopox** have similar presentations (fever followed by rash). Very few infect humans, including monkeypox (recently spread by prairie dogs), cowpox (cause "milker's nodules" on hands of dairy workers), and Orf (nodule on hands, arms, or face after exposure to ruminants)
- **Parapox** viruses are notable for molluscum contagiosum, the cause of umbilicated firm papules on the skin. May be more persistent in immunocompromised adults, and typically are treated with curettage or cryotherapy

Papillomaviruses

- Human papillomavirus (HPV) is ubiquitous infection causing benign and malignant tumors of skin and mucosal surfaces
- Over 100 "types," with types 6 and 11 most closely associated with anogenital warts ("condyloma acuminatum"), 16 and 18 linked to cervical cancer and respiratory polyps.
- Diagnosis: Visual exam (direct or colposcopic), Pap smear, and detection and typing of viral DNA by PCR
- Treatment: Local therapy (excision or cryotherapy). Vaccine under development may prevent infection with common types

POLYOMAVIRUSES

- BK and JC viruses are widespread in US and Western Europe (60% to 80% of population with serum antibodies)

- Latent infection may be present in the kidney, and **viuria is common** among immunosuppressed
- BK virus is the cause of hemorrhagic cystitis in transplant patients, while JC virus is the cause of primary multifocal leukoencephalopathy in patients with HIV
- Diagnosis: PCR
- Treatment: Cidofovir may be effective

MEASLES/MUMPS/RUBELLA

- All are diagnosed by serology, and treatment is supportive

Measles (Rubeola)

- Very infectious paramyxovirus spread via respiratory droplet
- Nearly 2 week incubation followed by constitutional symptoms, "classic" **cough, coryza,** and **Koplik's spots** (small, bluish granules on erythematous buccal mucosa)
- Erythematous maculopapular rash spread craniocaudally and may desquamate and involve palms/soles
- Complications: Pneumonia with secondary bacterial superinfection, encephalitis (may be chronic in subacute sclerosing panencephalitis)

Mumps

- Paramyxovirus acquired through nasopharyngeal contact with respiratory droplets or fomites leads to extended (2 to 4 week) incubation period
- Clinical illness heralded by **otalgia, parotid hypertrophy,** and **sialadenitis**, and may be followed by meningitis, encephalitis, or orchitis

Rubella (German Measles)

- Benign viral infection characterized by fever and maculopapular, nonconfluent craniocaudal rash. May occasionally be complicated by arthralgias
- Congenital infection may lead to fetal death and **congenital abnormalities** (hearing loss, heart disease, cognitive delay)

PARVOVIRUS

- Smallest DNA virus with widespread infection. 50% of adolescents and nearly all elderly persons have serum antibodies to parvovirus B19
- Spread among close contacts by respiratory droplets or blood

- Causes **erythema infectiosum** ("slapped cheek"), **arthritis, red cell aplasia/aplastic crisis,** and **hemophagocytic syndrome**
- Fetal infection may lead to **hydrops fetalis** or miscarriage (especially during first trimester)
- Diagnosis: PCR or serology
- Treatment: IV immunoglobulin (IVIG)

RABIES

- Causes fatal encephalitis, acquired through bite of infected mammals (dogs in the developing world, bats or raccoons more likely in developed countries)
- Risk of acquiring virus from rabid animal varies by type of exposure. Increased risk with more saliva, bites on face vs. extremities, unprotected skin vs. clothed
- **Incubation period** can be prolonged (up to 5 years) but most patients will develop symptoms in first 90 days
- Pain at wound site and constitutional symptoms is followed by neurologic symptoms (change in behavior, hallucinations, **autonomic dysfunction,** and **ascending flaccid paralysis**)
- Diagnosis: DFA of tissue from animal or infected human (especially from nape of neck biopsy)
- Treatment: Cleansing of wound and rabies vaccine immediately after exposure.
- Clinical disease **virtually always fatal**

FLAVIVIRUSES

- Heterogeneous group zoonotic/arthropod transmitted viruses
- Diagnosis for all is via serology (IgM during acute illness or IgG in convalescence) or PCR. No specific therapy

West Nile

- Rapidly emerging virus across US since 1999
- Transmitted from reservoirs in birds to humans via mosquitoes
- Majority of infections are without symptoms or with only fever and malaise, but most severe complications are neurological (encephalitis and **muscle weakness**)

Dengue

- Tropical, transmitted by *Aedes aegypti* (day-biting) mosquito
- Illness characterized by high fever, headache (often retro-orbital), myalgias/arthralgias, and rash

- Hemorrhagic fever or shock may occur shortly after resolution of fever. May be more common in persons previously exposed

Yellow Fever

- Endemic to sub-Saharan Africa and South America
- Transmitted by mosquito bites
- Symptoms range from mild constitutional to severe. Symptomatic patients likely to experience headache, altered mental status, icterus, and many have diffuse hemorrhage
- Preventable by vaccine, although vaccine may induce encephalitis among young infants or the elderly

Other Flaviviruses

- Japanese encephalitis: Fevers and altered mental status in Asian regions where mosquitoes interact with pigs and birds
- St. Louis encephalitis: Fevers and altered mental status, especially among the elderly. Seen in North, Central, and South America as well as the Caribbean
- Tick-borne encephalitis: Infection via *Ixodes* ticks in Europe and Asia among persons with outdoor exposure. Fever, may progress to altered mental status and paralysis

HEMORRHAGIC VIRUSES

- Group includes Filoviridae (Ebola and Marburg viruses), Bunyaviridae (Hantavirus), and Arenaviridae (Lassa virus)

Filoviridae

- Acquired through contact with nonhuman primates in Africa
- Fevers and myalgias are followed by maculopapular rash, after which between 10% and 50% will develop disseminated intravascular coagulation
- Diagnosis: Serology (IgM early) or PCR
- Treatment: Supportive

Bunyaviridae

- Rift Valley fever: Via *Aedes* mosquitoes in sub-Saharan Africa
- Crimean-Congo hemorrhagic fever: Transmitted by ticks in Southwest Asia, Middle East, and Africa

- Hantavirus: Transmitted by wild rodents. Two types: Asian strains, which cause fever and renal failure, and North American strains, which cause fever and pulmonary edema

Arenaviruses

- Transmitted to humans via contact with rodents
- Endemic to Africa and South America

RETROVIRUSES

- Unique use of reverse transcriptase to make DNA from RNA
- Divided broadly into oncoviruses (human T cell lymphotropic virus 1 and 2 [HTLV-1 and -2]) and lentiviruses (HIV; see Chapter 16)
- Transmitted via sexual or parenteral contact

HTLV-1 and -2

- HTLV-1 found in geographic pockets in the Caribbean, Central/South America, West Africa, Japan, Australia, and New Zealand. HTLV-2 is endemic among Native Americans and some intravenous drug users
- HTLV-1 causes adult T cell leukemia/lymphoma, leading to skin and bone involvement. It also causes tropical spastic paresis, which manifests as lower extremity motor weakness and spasms due to demyelination of the thoracic spinal cord
- HTLV-2 has been weakly associated with hairy cell leukemia and mycosis fungoides
- Diagnosis: Serology
- Treatment: Steroids, interferon-α, zidovudine

3

Antimicrobial Agents

Timothy H. Dellit, MD

■ Mechanisms of Action

- Inhibit cell wall synthesis
  - Bind to **penicillin binding proteins** (PBP) and inhibit peptidoglycan cross-linking
    - Penicillins, cephalosporins, carbapenems, monobactams
  - Bind to D-alanyl-D-alanine precursors, preventing incorporation into cell wall
    - Vancomycin
- Target cell membrane
  - Depolarization of bacterial cell membrane
    - Daptomycin
- Inhibit protein synthesis
  - Bind to 30S ribosomal subunit
    - Aminoglycosides, tetracyclines
  - Bind to 50S ribosomal subunit
    - Chloramphenicol, clindamycin, ketolides, macrolides, streptogramins
  - Prevents the formation of the 70S initiation complex
    - Linezolid
- Inhibit or damage nucleic acids
  - Inhibit DNA gyrase and topoisomerase IV
    - Fluoroquinolones
  - Intracellular reduction leading to DNA damage
    - Metronidazole, nitrofurantoin
  - Inhibit DNA-dependent RNA polymerase
    - Rifampin
- Anti-metabolites
  - Inhibit folic acid metabolism
    - Sulfonamides, trimethoprim

■ General Mechanisms of Resistance

- Alteration of antimicrobial activity
  - Bacterial production of **beta-lactamases,** which inactivate beta-lactam antibiotics, is a common mechanism, particularly in gram-negative organisms and *Staphylococcus aureus*
    - This has led to the combination of a beta-lactamase inhibitor with a beta-lactam antibiotic: Amoxicillin-clavulanate,

ampicillin-sulbactam, piperacillin-tazobactam, ticarcillin-clavulanate
- Alteration of target site
  - **Alteration of PBP** leads to penicillin-resistant *Streptococcus pneumoniae*
- Alteration of **drug permeability** into and/or efflux out of the bacterial cell
  - Quinupristin-dalfopristin inactive against *Enterococcus faecalis* due to intrinsic efflux of dalfopristin

■ Clinical Implications of Resistance

- *Streptococcus pyogenes* (group A *Streptococcus*)
  - Uniformly **susceptible to penicillin**
  - Increasing resistance to macrolides associated with increased use, roughly 5% nationally
- *Streptococcus pneumoniae*
  - Nationally, 35% nonsusceptible to penicillin (13% intermediate, 22% resistant) (Table 3-1)
- *S. aureus*
  - Methicillin-resistant *S. aureus* (MRSA) has an alternative target encoded by the *mecA* gene called PBP 2a that has low affinity for beta-lactams
    - Resistant to all beta-lactams including cephalosporins and carbapenems
    - **Vancomycin remains the "gold standard" for MRSA** with other potential options based on severity of infection and local susceptibility patterns (recommend discussing with attending or infectious disease service before using alternative agent)
  - Vancomycin resistance is rare, but has been reported
- *Enterococcus*
  - Vancomycin-resistant *Enterococcus* (VRE) has alternative cell wall precursors with low affinity for vancomycin (*vanA* gene encodes D-Ala-D-Lac instead of D-Ala-D-Ala)
    - Treatment options for VRE include **linezolid** or **quinupristin/dalfopristin**, although *E. faecalis* is resistant to the latter

■ TABLE 3-1 Drug Resistance Among Pneumococcal Isolates	
Antimicrobial Agent	**Resistance (%)**
Macrolide	31
TMP/SMX	20–36
Tetracycline	8–17
Fluoroquinolones	2

- *E. coli* and urinary tract infections
  - **Ampicillin resistance** roughly 40%
  - Geographic variation in resistance to TMP/SMX
    - If regional resistance to TMP/SMX ≥ 20%, an alternative agent such as a fluoroquinolone should be considered
- *Neisseria gonorrhoeae*
  - Parenteral ceftriaxone or PO cefpodoxime is preferred therapy due to increasing fluoroquinolone resistance
- AmpC beta-lactamases and SPICE organisms
  - Monotherapy with a third generation cephalosporin may be associated with the induction of ampC beta-lactamase in SPICE organisms
    - *Serratia, Pseudomonas, Providencia,* indole-positive *Proteus, Citrobacter, Enterobacter, Morganella*
- Extended spectrum beta-lactamases (ESBLs)
  - Most common with *Klebsiella* and *E. coli*, though a minority of strains
  - A carbapenem is the drug of choice in infections due to an ESBL-producing organism

■ **Spectrum of Antibiotic Activity**

- See Tables 3-2 and 3-3

TABLE 3-2 Spectrum of Antibiotic Activity

	Penicillin	Ampicillin/ Amoxicillin	Amp/Sulb, Amox/Clav	Oxacillin	Pip/Tazo Ticar/Clav	Cefazolin (1st Gen)	Cefuroxime (2nd Gen)	Ceftriaxone (3rd Gen)	Ceftazidime (3rd Gen)	Cefepime (4th Gen)	Carbapenem[a]	Aztreonam
Strep group A,B,C,G	++	++	++	++	++	++	++	++	+	++	++	−
S. pneumoniae	+[b]	+	+	+	+	+	+	++	+	++	++	−
Enterococcus	+	++	++	−	+/−[c]	−	−	−	−	−	+	−
S. aureus	−	−	+	++	++	++	+	++	+/−	++	++	−
MRSA	−	−	−	−	−	−	−	−	−	−	−	−
Moraxella/ H. influenzae	−	+/−[d]	++	−	++	+	+	++	++	++	++	++
E. coli/ K. pneumoniae	−	+/−	++	−	++	+	+	++	++	++	++	++
P. aeruginosa	−	−	−	−	++	−	−	−	++	++	++	++
SPICE[e]	−	−	−	−	++	−	−	++	++	++	++	++
S. maltophilia	−	−	−	−	+[f]	−	−	−	−	−	−	−
Atypicals[g]	−	−	−	−	−	−	−	−	−	−	−	−
Anaerobes (Mouth)	+	++	++	−	++	−	−	+	−	−	++	−
Anaerobes (Gut)	−	−	++	−	++	−	−	+	−	+/−	++	−
Strep group A,B,C,G	++	++	++	+[i]	++	++	++	+	+	+	++	−
S. pneumoniae	++	++	++	+[j]	++	+	+	+	+	+/−	++	−

(Continued)

TABLE 3-2 Continued

	Vancomycin	Linezolid	Quinupristin-dalfopristin	Daptomycin	Clindamycin	Metronidazole	Macrolides	Ketolides	TMP/SMX	Tetracyclines	Fluoroquinolones[h]	Aminoglycosides[h]
Enterococcus	++	++	++[i]	++	−	−	−	−	−	−	+/−	−[k]
S. aureus	++	++	++	++	++	−	+	+	+	+	+	−[k]
MRSA	++	++	++	++	+[l]	−	−	−	+[l]	+[l]	−[l]	−
Moraxella/ H.influenzae	−	−	−	−	−	−	+	+	+	+	++	++
E.coli[i]	−	−	−	−	−	−	−	−	+	+/−	++	++
K.pneumoniae	−	−	−	−	−	−	−	−	−	−	++	++
P.aeruginosa	−	−	−	−	−	−	−	−	−	−	++	++
SPICE[e]	−	−	−	−	−	−	−	−	−	−	++	++
S.maltophilia	−	−	−	−	−	−	−	−	+	−	+/−	−
Atypicals[g]	−	−	−	−	−	−	+	+	−	+	++	−
Anaerobes (Mouth)	−	+	+	−	++	++	−	−	−	−	+/−	−
Anaerobes (Gut)	−	−	−	−	++	++	−	−	−	−	+/−	−

aErtapenem is not active against Pseudomonas or Acinetobacter. bIntermediate 13%, resistant 22%. cPip/tazo is more active. dFrequently resistant due to beta-lactamase production. eSerratia, Providencia, indole-positive Proteus, Citrobacter, Enterobacter, and Morganella. fTicar/clav has activity. gChlamydia, Legionella, Mycoplasma. hSee Table 3.3 for selected properties of fluoroquinolones. iNot active against E. faecalis. jNot effective in the treatment of pneumonia. kUsed for synergy in endocarditis. lDependent on local susceptibilities and severity of infection.

Abbreviations: ++, highly active; +, moderately active; may use if susceptible; +/−, minimally active, would not use as first line agent;−, very poorly or not active; Amox/Clav, amoxicillin–clavulanate; Amp/Sulb, ampicillin–sulbactam; MRSA, methicillin-resistant S. aureus; Pip/Tazo, piperacillin–tazobactam; Ticar/Clav, ticarcillin-clavulanate

■ TABLE 3-3   Selected Properties of Fluoroquinolones

Fluoroquinolone	Distinguishing Characteristics
Ciprofloxacin	Most active fluoroquinolone against *P. aeruginosa*
Enoxacin	Similar to norfloxacin, but more side effects
Gatifloxacin	Enhanced activity against *S. pneumoniae*, atypicals, anaerobes
Gemifloxacin	Enhanced activity against *S. pneumoniae*, atypicals, anaerobes
Levofloxacin	Moderately active against *S. pneumoniae* and *P. aeruginosa*
Lomefloxacin	Less active against *S. pneumoniae*, streptococci, atypicals; phototoxicity
Moxifloxacin	Enhanced activity against *S. pneumoniae*, atypicals, anaerobes
Norfloxacin	Intestinal and genitourinary infections only
Ofloxacin	Same spectrum as levofloxacin
Trovafloxacin	Active against *S. pneumoniae*, *P. aeruginosa*, and anaerobes; serious hepatotoxicity reported, no longer available

Notes:

Earlier fluoroquinolones such as ciprofloxacin and levofloxacin bind primarily to either DNA gyrase (gram-negative organisms) or to topoisomerase IV (gram-positive organisms). The newer fluoroquinolones (gatifloxacin, gemifloxacin, and moxifloxacin) bind equivalently to both targets. This would imply that concurrent mutations in both target enzymes would be required for resistance to develop.

Fluoroquinolones demonstrate concentration-dependent killing with the ratio of area under the curve (AUC) to the minimal inhibitory concentration (MIC) best correlated with clinical efficacy. For *S. pneumoniae*, these ratios are best for the newer fluoroquinolones, particularly moxifloxacin.

These two concepts have led to the argument favoring the newer fluoroquinolones such as moxifloxacin over levofloxacin for community-acquired pneumonia, if a fluoroquinolone is to be used.

Antifungal Agents

Theoklis E. Zaoutis, MD, MSCE

ANTIFUNGAL AGENTS USED FOR TREATMENT OF INVASIVE FUNGAL INFECTIONS

Polyenes

■ **Agents**

- Amphotericin B deoxycholate
- Lipid formulations of amphotericin B (less nephrotoxic)
  - Amphotericin B lipid complex
  - Amphotericin B cholesteryl sulfate
  - Liposomal amphotericin B

■ **Mechanism of Action**

- Binds to the sterol ergosterol in the fungal **cell membrane** and causes changes in cell permeability leading to cell lysis and death

■ **Antifungal Activity** (Tables 4-1, 4-2, and 4-3)

- Broad-spectrum of antifungal activity against most pathogenic fungi, both yeasts and molds, in humans
- *Candida* spp are rarely resistant, with the exception of *C. lusitaniae*
- *Aspergillus terreus, Trichosporon beiglelli, Fusarium* spp, *Pseudallescheria boydii, Scedosporium prolificans,* and other dematiaceous fungi may be resistant to amphotericin B
- Lipid formulations of amphotericin B have similar therapeutic activity to conventional amphotericin B deoxycholate

■ **Adverse Effects**

- **Nephrotoxicity** associated with azotemia and **wasting of potassium and magnesium** is common and usually reversible. However, on occasion can lead to renal failure and need for dialysis
- Nephrotoxicity is exacerbated by concomitant use of other nephrotoxic agents
- **Infusion-related reactions** such as fever, rigors, chills, myalgias, arthralgias, vomiting, and headaches are commonly seen in patients receiving amphotericin B, and these reactions can lead to discontinuation of therapy

■ TABLE 4-1 Antifungal Susceptibilities Against *Candida* Species and *Cryptococcus Neoformans*

Yeasts	Amphotericin	Fluconazole	Voriconazole	Caspofungin	Itraconazole	5-FC[a]
C. albicans	S	S	S	S	S	S
C. tropicalis	S	S	S	S	S	S
C. parapsilosis	S	S	S	S	S	S
C. glabrata	S-I	DDS-R	S	S	DDS-R	S
C. krusei	S-I	R	S	S	DDS-R	I-R
C. lusitaniae	R	S	S	S	S	S
Cryptococcus neoformans[b]	S	S	S	R	S	S

[a] 5-FC is not used as monotherapy, because of the rapid development of resistance

[b] Treatment recommendations and potential first-line agents vary by organism and clinical manifestation of infection. Invasive candidiasis: amphotericin, fluconazole, and caspofungin; CNS or serious cryptococcal infections: amphotericin in combination with 5-FC; mild to moderate pulmonary cryptococcal infections: amphotericin B, itraconazole, or fluconazole

Abbreviations: DDS, dose-dependant susceptible; I, intermediate; R, resistant; S, susceptible

■ TABLE 4-2 Antifungal Activity Against Clinically Encountered Dimorphic Fungi

Mycosis	Drug of Choice[a]	Alternative Agents[b]
Histoplasma capsulatum	Amphotericin and/or itraconazole	Fluconazole
Coccidioides immitis	Amphotericin, itraconazole, fluconazole, ketoconazole	—
Blastomycosis dermatitidis	Amphotericin and/or itraconazole	Fluconazole and ketoconazole
Sporothrix schenckii	Amphotericin and/or itraconazole	Fluconazole

[a] Treatment recommendation may depend on the clinical manifestation of infection
[b] Alternative azole agents in patients unable to tolerate itraconazole

■ TABLE 4-3 Antifungal Activity Against Clinically Encountered Molds

Mycosis	Drug of Choice	Alternative Agents
Aspergillus spp	Voriconazole or amphotericin	Caspofungin[a]
Fusarium or alternaria[b]	Amphotericin	Voriconazole
Zycomycetes (mucormycosis)	Amphotericin	—
Malassezia furfur (systemic infection)	Fluconazole	Itraconazole

[a] Caspofungin is indicated for the treatment of invasive aspergillosis in patients who are refractory to or intolerant of other therapies
[b] Resistant to 5-FC, ketoconazole, fluconazole, echinocandins, miconazole, and itraconazole

• Lipid formulations of amphotericin B are associated with reduced nephrotoxicity and infusion-related side effects
• Mild increases in transaminases, bilirubin, and alkaline phosphatase have been observed with all the lipid formulations of amphotericin B

Triazoles

■ Agents

• First generation: Fluconazole, itraconazole, ketoconazole
• Second generation: Voriconazole, posaconazole,* ravuconazole* (*FDA approval pending)

■ Mechanism of Action

• Inhibits cytochrome P-450 enzymes used in the synthesis of the fungal **cell membrane**

■ **Antifungal Activity** (see Tables 4-1, 4-2, and 4-3)

• Fluconazole and itraconazole are active against **Candida** spp but have decreased activity against C. *glabrata* and C. *tropicalis,* and are not active against C. *krusei*

• Both agents are active against **Cryptococcus neoformans** and T. *beiglii*

• Fluconazole is not active against molds

• Itraconazole is active against *Aspergillus* spp and dematiaceous molds but is inactive against *Fusarium* spp. and zygomycetes

• Both agents are active against **dimorphic fungi** such as *Histoplasma capsulatum, Coccidioides immitis, Blastomyces dermatidis, Paracoccidioides brasiliensis,* and *Sporothrix schenkii*

• The second-generation triazole agents have broader activity and are active against **Aspergillus spp,** *Fusarium,* and other hyaline and dematiaceous molds

■ **Adverse Effects**

• Significant drug-drug interactions occur secondary to interaction with CYP-450 enzyme system. Triazoles interfere with anticonvulsant medications, tacrolimus, cyclosporin A, rifampin, clarithromycin, several of the antiretroviral agents, and many other medications

• All the triazoles are generally well tolerated but occasionally can cause mild elevations in **liver transaminases**

• Itraconazole has significant **gastrointestinal disturbances** associated with the oral formulation

• Voriconazole use has been associated with transient **visual disturbances**

Echinocandins

■ **Agents**

• Caspofungin
• Micafungin
• Anidulafungin (FDA approval pending)

■ **Mechanism of Action**

• Cyclic lipopeptide structure that inhibits 1,3 β-D-glucan synthase. Glucan is the major component of the **fungal cell wall**

■ **Antifungal Activity** (see Tables 4-1 and 4-3)

• Potent broad-spectrum fungicidal activity against **Candida spp.** No cross-resistance seen to amphotericin B or azole-resistant *Candida* spp

• Potent inhibitory activity against **Aspergillus spp**

- Inactive against *C. neoformans, T. beiglii,* zygomycetes, and hyalohypomycetes
- Active against *Pneumocystis carinii*

■ Adverse Reactions

- Generally well tolerated
- Most common side effects seen include **fever,** increased **liver transaminases,** phlebitis, nausea, and headache
- Caspofungin should be used with caution in patients receiving **cyclosporine** because of potential interaction leading to increased caspofungin levels. The drug interaction is not mediated by the CYP 450 enzyme system

Flucytosine

■ Agent

- 5-FC

■ Mechanism of Action

- Inhibits **RNA and DNA synthesis**

■ Antifungal Activity (see Table 4-1)

- Essentially limited to **Candida spp, C. neoformans**
- No activity against *Aspergillus* spp and other molds
- Resistance to 5-FC is rapidly acquired and therefore it is not given as a single agent
- Most commonly used in combination with amphotericin B or fluconazole for the treatment of **cryptococcal meningitis** or deep-tissue infections with **Candida** spp

■ Adverse Reactions

- Serious side effects include **bone marrow suppression** (usually reversible)
- Common adverse effects include **gastrointestinal intolerance** and elevations in **liver transaminases**

ANTIFUNGALS USED FOR TREATMENT OF SKIN AND MUCOSAL FUNGAL INFECTIONS

Griseofulvin

■ Agent

- Griseofulvin

■ Mechanism of Action
- Interferes with fungal **microtubule formation**

■ Antifungal Activity
- Active against dermatophytes including *Microsporon*, *Epidermophyton*, and *Trichophyton*
- Most commonly used for the treatment of **tinea capitis** and refractory **tinea corporis**

■ Adverse Affects
- Most common side effects are **headache** and **gastrointestinal disturbances**
- Can also cause rash and is contraindicated in patients with hepatic failure
- Can produce a **disulfiram reaction** when taken concurrently with alcohol
- Contraindicated in pregnant women
- Enhances the clearance of oral contraceptives, cyclosporine, theophylline, aspirin, and warfarin

Allylamines

■ Agents
- Terbinafine
- Naftine

■ Mechanism of Action
- Inhibits the biosynthesis of fungal **ergosterol** in the fungal cell membrane

■ Antifungal Activity
- Potent activity against **dermatophytes**
- Also active against *Aspergillus*, *Fusarium*, dematiaceous and dimorphic fungi, and *P. carinii*, but has not been effective for treatment of infections caused by these organisms in animal models
- Indicated for the topical or oral treatment of **skin and nail infections** caused by dermatophytes and possibly for cutaneous sporotrichosis

■ Adverse Effects
- Generally well tolerated
- Primary adverse effects are **gastrointestinal upset and skin** reactions
- Rarely can cause hepatitis and liver failure

Imidazoles

■ Agents

- Clotrimazole (topical only)
- Miconazole (topical only)
- Ketoconazole

■ Mechanism of Action

- Inhibits cytochrome P-450 enzymes used in the synthesis of the **fungal cell membrane**

■ Antifungal Activity

- Active against **oropharyngeal** and **vulvovaginal candidiasis** and *Candida* dermatitis
- Active against tinea versicolor

■ Adverse Effects

- Ketoconazole, when given orally can cause nausea, vomiting, abdominal pain, headache
- Rashes, pruritus, and urticaria

Polyenes

■ Agent

- Nystatin

■ Mechanism of Action

- Binds to the sterol ergosterol in the **fungal cell membrane** and causes changes in cell permeability leading to cell lysis and death

■ Antifungal Activity

- Used for topical treatment of oral, gastrointestinal, esophageal, and genital candidiasis
- A liposomal IV formulation for the treatment of systemic fungal infections is in development

■ Adverse Effects

- Topical nystatin can cause local skin irritation
- Oral nystatin can cause nausea, vomiting, and diarrhea

Antiviral Agents Including Antiretrovirals

George A. Diaz, MD

ANTIVIRAL AGENTS

Influenza Antivirals

■ **Amantadine and Rimantadine** (differ by an extra ethyl group)
- Mechanisms of action
  - Inhibition of ion channel function of M2 protein, which **blocks viral uncoating** during endocytosis at low concentrations
  - At higher lysosomal concentrations, **viral fusion is inhibited**
- Mechanism of resistance: Single amino acid change in transmembrane region of M2 protein, occurs in 30% of isolates by day 5 of therapy
- Spectrum of activity:
  - **Influenza A** (not B at normal doses), respiratory syncytial virus (RSV)
  - At high in vitro concentrations: Parainfluenza, influenza B, rubella, hepatitis C, and dengue

■ **Oseltamivir and Zanamivir**
- Mechanism of action: Neuraminidase inhibitors
  - **Prevents release of virus from infected cells** by allowing the persistence of the natural target for viral hemagglutinin
- Mechanism of resistance: Mutations in either viral neuraminidase or hemagglutinin
- Spectrum of activity: **Influenza A and B**

■ **Ribavirin**
- Mechanism of action: **Guanosine analog**
  - Not fully understood, but likely alters nucleotide pools and mRNA production
- Mechanism of resistance: Occurs only in Sindbis virus, by an unknown mechanism
- Spectrum of activity: **RSV** in children, **chronic hepatitis C** infection in conjunction with pegylated interferon (IFN), severe influenza infections, Lassa fever, and hemorrhagic fevers (Argentine, Sabia,

Bolivian, Crimean Congo). Possibly useful in severe parainfluenza, measles, vaccinia, adenovirus infections

Herpesvirus Antivirals

■ Cidofovir

- Mechanism of action: Once phosphorylated, competitively **inhibits DNA polymerase** and slows chain elongation
- Mechanism of resistance: DNA polymerase mutations combined with UL97 mutation (confers high-level ganciclovir resistance) may be cross-resistant to cidofovir. Other DNA polymerase mutations may cause resistance
- Spectrum of activity: **Cytomegalovirus (CMV), varicella zoster virus (VZV), Epstein-Barr virus (EBV), human herpesvirus 6 (HHV-6), HHV-8, papillomaviruses, poxviruses, adenoviruses**

■ Fomivirsen

- Mechanism of action: A 21-nucleotide DNA sequence that is complementary to mRNA transcript of Major Immediate Early region 2 of CMV
- Mechanism of resistance: Unknown
- Spectrum of activity: Intravitreal injection in the treatment of **CMV retinitis**

■ Foscarnet

- Mechanism of action: **Directly inhibits viral DNA polymerase, as well as HIV reverse transcriptase**
- Mechanism of resistance: Point mutations in DNA polymerase
- Spectrum of activity: **CMV, herpes simplex virus 1 (HSV-1) and -2, VZV, EBV, HHV-8**

■ Acyclovir and Valacyclovir

- Valacyclovir is L-valyl ester prodrug of acyclovir
- Mechanism of action: Activated by viral thymidine kinase and **competitively inhibits viral DNA polymerase** and terminates DNA chain
- Mechanisms of resistance
  - Absent or low levels of viral thymidine kinase
  - Alteration in thymidine kinase specificity to exclude phosphorylation of acyclovir
  - Altered viral DNA polymerase
- Spectrum of activity: **HSV-1 and -2, VZV, CMV, EBV**

■ Penciclovir and Famciclovir

- Famciclovir is diacetyl ester of 6-deoxypenciclovir
- Mechanism of action: Competitive inhibitor of DNA polymerase, also depends on viral thymidine kinase for activity

- Mechanism of resistance: Thymidine kinase-deficient strains
- Spectrum of activity: **HSV, VZV, hepatitis B virus,** and possibly EBV

■ Ganciclovir and Valganciclovir

- Mechanism of action: Acyclic guanoside that competitively **inhibits DNA polymerase. It depends on viral thymidine kinase in HSV and VZV** and the UL97 product in CMV
- Mechanism of resistance: UL97 mutation in CMV and other DNA polymerase mutations
- Spectrum of activity: **CMV, HSV-1 and -2, EBV, and HHV-6**

■ Idoxuridine

- Mechanism of action: **Thymidine analog,** inhibits both viral and cellular DNA synthesis
- Mechanism of resistance: Unknown
- Spectrum of activity: **HSV keratitis,** possibly VZV, human papilloma virus, and poxviruses

■ Trifluridine

- Mechanism of action: Trifluridine monophosphate irreversibly inhibits thymidylate synthetase, and trifluridine triphosphate inhibits viral and cellular DNA polymerases
- Mechanism of resistance: Unknown
- Spectrum of activity: HSV keratitis, HSV-1 and -2, CMV, vaccinia, and adenoviruses

■ Vidarabine

- Mechanism of action: Analog of adenosine that inhibits viral DNA synthesis through its 5′-triphosphorylated metabolite, which competitively inhibits the activity of viral and cellular DNA polymerases
- Mechanism of resistance: Mutations in viral DNA polymerase are seen in vitro, but not in vivo
- Spectrum of activity: HSV keratitis, HSV-1 and -2, VZV, EBV, poxviruses, rhabdoviruses, and RNA tumor viruses, but **currently available only as topical agent**

ANTIRETROVIRAL AGENTS (see also Chapter 16)

- Initial regimens should be individualized considering comorbid conditions, medication interactions, and patient's lifestyle and views on therapy

- Treatment of HIV is constantly evolving, but current recommendations suggest initiating therapy using three-drug regimens consisting of two nucleoside reverse transcriptase inhibitors (NRTIs) such as AZT/3TC (Combivir), abacavir (ABC) with lamivudine (3TC), or tenofovir (TNF) with 3TC, and a non-nucleoside reverse transcriptase inhibitor (NNRTI) such as efavirenz (EFV) or a protease inhibitor (PI) such as ritonavir (RTV)-boosted lopinavir (LPV)
- Less commonly used antiretrovirals include zalcitabine (ddC), delaviridine (DLV), and full-dose RTV (although RTV is often used at lower boosting doses in conjunction with other PIs)
- Many side effects and drug interactions known. The following antiretrovirals should not be combined: zidovudine (AZT) and stavudine (d4T) (antagonism), 3TC and emtricitabine (FTC) (similar drugs), atazanavir (ATV) and indinavir (IDV) (hyperbilirubinemia), fosamprenavir (F-APV) and amprenavir (APV) (similar drugs), d4T and didanosine (ddI) (fatal lactic acidosis, pancreatitis, peripheral neuropathy)

Nucleoside Reverse Transcriptase Inhibitors (NRTIs)

■ **ABC, Combivir, ddI, FTC, 3TC, d4T, Trizivir (ABC/AZT/3TC), AZT, ddC**

- Mechanism of action: Analogs of nucleosides, are converted to triphosphate forms by cellular kinases, and, via the DNA polymerase function of the viral reverse transcriptase, are incorporated into the growing DNA chain, leading to chain termination due to the absence of a 3′-hydroxyl group needed to form a phosphodiester bond with the incoming nucleotide
- Mechanisms of resistance (an expanding number of mutations are being identified)
  - Mutations that help reverse transcriptase prevent NRTI incorporation in the growing DNA strand, preventing chain termination
  - Mutations that cause the hydrolytic removal of the chain-terminating NRTI, resulting in continued DNA synthesis
- Spectrum of activity: **HIV-1, HIV-2, and human T lymphotropic virus type 1 (HTLV-1).** Additionally, lamivudine is used in combination with an IFN to treat hepatitis B
- Potential side effects
  - AZT: Bone marrow suppression, myopathy, macrocytosis
  - d4T and ddI: Peripheral neuropathy, pancreatitis
  - All NRTIs, especially d4T and ddI rarely associated with life-threatening lactic acidosis (nausea, vomiting, abdominal pain, weight loss, fatigue) due to mitochondrial toxicity

Nucleotide Reverse Transcriptase Inhibitor (NtRTI)

■ TNF

- Mechanism of action: Differs from NRTIs by having a phosphate group in the parent molecule thus requiring only diphosphorylation to be converted to an active compound
- Mechanism of resistance: Classically a K65R mutation, but other mechanisms are the same as for NRTI
- Spectrum of activity: **HIV-1, HIV-2 and hepatitis B virus**

Non-Nucleoside Reverse Transcriptase Inhibitors (NNRTIs)

■ EFV, nevirapine (NVP), DLV

- Mechanism of action: Noncompetitively bind near the active site of the reverse transcriptase, disrupting the catalytic aspartate residues of the polymerase binding sites and resulting in an inactive state. Does not require cellular activation
- Mechanism of resistance: Multiple mutations, but K103N is the most commonly seen mutation, which results in resistance to all NNRTIs
- Spectrum of activity: **HIV-1,** except group O; inactive against HIV-2
- Potential side effects
  - NVP: Life-threatening hypersensitivity reaction
  - EFV: CNS symptoms, vivid dreams

Protease Inhibitors

■ APV, ATV, F-APV, IDV, LPV/RTV, RT, saquinavir (Fortovase [SQV-soft gel capsule] or Invirase [SQV-hard gel capsule]), nelfinavir (NFV or NLF)

- Mechanism of action: Inactivates the HIV protease responsible for the generation of reverse transcriptase, integrase, protease, matrix, capsid, nucleocapsid, and p6 proteins. This results in the generation of an immature defective virus
- Mechanism of resistance: Multiple mutations
- Spectrum of activity: **HIV-1 and -2**
- Common side effects
  - All PIs: Hyperglycemia, **central fat accumulation,** peripheral fat wasting, **elevated cholesterol and triglyceride levels**
  - Several PIs associated with GI intolerance
  - IOV: Nephrolithiasis and hyperbilirubinemia
  - NFV: Diarrhea
  - ATV may have less impact on lipids than other PIs

Fusion Inhibitor

■ Enfuvirtide (ENF/T-20)

- Mechanism of action: Synthetic peptide, binds HR1 site in the gp41 subunit of the envelope glycoprotein preventing viral fusion and entry into CD4+ cell
- Mechanism of resistance: Mutations in positions 36 and 45 of gp41 result in resistance
- Spectrum of activity: HIV-1
- Potential side effect: Given as a subcutaneous injection, local site reactions are common even when rotating sites

INTERFERONS

- Mechanism of action: Cytokines that signal through IFN receptors, which activates the JAK/STAT signaling pathway, which leads to the activation of 100 IFN-related genes and the generation of many proteins whose antiviral properties include inhibiting viral penetration, uncoating, transcription, translation, and assembly of new virions
- Mechanism of resistance: Variety of viruses have IFN-blocking properties
- Spectrum of activity: Condyloma acuminatum, hepatitis B virus, hepatitis C virus, Kaposi's sarcoma
- Pegylated IFN shown to be superior for treatment of hepatitis C

6 Ophthalmologic Infections

Erich H.P. Braun, MD

Before any intervention or consult request, always document the patient's vision (ideally with patient's glasses) and pupillary exam, and determine any prior eye surgery (i.e., cataract surgery) or contact lens use.

Infectious Conjunctivitis

Red, irritated conjunctiva with clear or mucopurulent discharge, usually without significant visual changes

■ Epidemiology

- Viral conjunctivitis may be highly contagious via direct contact or fomites
- *Neisseria gonorrhoeae:* More common in sexually active adults
- *Chlamydia trachomatis:* **Spread by the 4 Fs** (fingers, fomites, flies, and fornication). It is the leading cause of preventable blindness worldwide

■ Risk Factors

- Sick contacts or direct hand-eye contact with pathogens
- Prior or concurrent **herpetic infection**
- Preexisting eye conditions: Dry eye, foreign bodies, trichiasis, nasolacrimal duct obstruction

■ Etiology (Table 6-1)

- Viral: **Adenovirus,** enteroviruses, Newcastle disease, influenza, measles, mumps, molluscum, HSV
- Common bacterial: *Streptococcus pneumoniae, Staphylococcus aureus, Haemophilus influenzae*
- Other bacterial: **N. gonorrhoeae,** *Neisseria meningitidis,* C. *trachomatis* (common in developing countries), *Moraxella catarrhalis, Proteus* spp, Enterobacteriaceae, *Pseudomonas aeruginosa* (intensive care unit patients), *Bartonella henselae* (Parinaud oculoglandular syndrome; also caused by *Francisella tularensis* and *Mycobacteria*)
- Other: Syphilis

■ **Pathogenesis**

- Bacterial or viral overgrowth and infiltration of the conjunctival epithelium and/or substantia propria with inflammation

■ **History/Physical Exam** (Table 6-1)

- Obtain ocular and immune status history
- Document **visual acuity** and pupillary exam
- Perform **eyelid eversion** to detect foreign bodies
- Viral: Red, pruritic, uncomfortable eye with clear discharge, erythematous/edematous eyelids, palpable preauricular nodes, may have small subconjunctival hemorrhages, contact with other symptomatic person, **contralateral eye involved within 2–4 days**
- Bacterial: Red, uncomfortable eye with mucopurulent discharge, foreign body sensation, papillary reaction, membranes or pseudomembranes on the tarsal conjunctiva, chemosis (edema of the conjunctiva)
- **Danger signs** that warrant immediate ophthalmology consult: Corneal opacity or hypesthesia, corneal dendritiform lesions with fluorescein staining, and marked photophobia

■ **Additional Studies**

- Additional studies depend on suspected etiology (see Table 6-1)

■ **Differential Diagnosis**

- Allergic conjunctivitis, dry eye syndrome, exposure, trauma, chemical exposure, contact lens-related irritation, keratitis, pterigium, blepharitis, pediculosis, molluscum contagiosum, ocular rosacea, acute glaucoma, uveitis, autoimmune disorders (e.g., Sjogren's, graft versus host), Stevens-Johnson, ocular cicatricial pemphigoid, episcleritis, scleritis, toxic medicamentosa, vascular abnormality, vitamin A deficiency, subconjunctival hemorrhage

■ **Management** (Table 6-1)

- Most viral and bacterial conjunctivitis will **resolve without treatment** in 7–14 days. **Consult ophthalmology if** (1) suspected HSV, gonococcal, or *P. aeruginosa* conjunctivitis; (2) corneal involvement; (3) tarsal membranes present; (4) any danger signs present (see above)
- Symptomatic relief with cold compresses PRN, artificial tears four to eight times daily, nephazoline/pheniramine drops four times daily
- Avoid topical steroid therapy unless recommended by an ophthalmologist

■ TABLE 6-1   Infectious Conjunctivitis

Organism	Ocular Signs/Symptoms	Evaluation*	Treatment	Other
Adenovirus	Itchy, watery, mucus discharge, lid erythema/edema, pinpoint sub-conjunctival blood, preauricular node, subepithelial infiltrates	None routinely indicated	May peel membrane or pseudomembrane Consider topical steroid only after ophthalmology consult	Highly contagious for 10–12 days after onset (There's a reason this is called "epidemic keratoconjunctivitis")
Bacterial (other than *Neisseria* spp)	Foreign body sensation (usually not pruritic), conjunctival papillae, purulent discharge, chemosis	Gram stain and bacterial culture: necessary only in severe cases. If sent, include cultures on blood and chocolate agar (for *Neisseria* spp)	Trimethoprim/polymyxin, ofloxacin or ciprofloxacin drops or bacitracin ophthalmic ointment for 5–7 days	Follow up every 2–5 days; adjust treatment based on culture results
C. trachomatis	Tarsal or limbal follicles, preauricular node, stringy mucus discharge, may have scarring, vascular limbal pannus Trachoma may have trichiasis, entropion, corneal opacification	Giemsa stain: Intracytoplasmic inclusions Chlamydial immunofluorescence and/or cultures	Oral doxycycline, erythromycin, or clarithromycin for 3–6 weeks Erythromycin ophthalmic ointment for 3–6 weeks	Inquire about STDs
HSV	Clear or mucoid discharge, photophobia, conjunctival follicles, chemosis, ±lid lesions, unilateral preauricular lymph node	Giemsa stain: Multinucleated giant cells HSV culture or ELISA	Trifluoridine 1% or vidarabine 3% ophthalmic ointment five times per day Erythromycin or bacitracin ophthalmic ointment to lid lesions twice daily to prevent bacterial super infection	Requires ophthalmology evaluation to exclude corneal involvement (keratitis; see Table 6-2)

(Continued)

■ TABLE 6-1	Continued			
Organism	Ocular Signs/Symptoms	Evaluation*	Treatment	Other
Neisseria spp	**Hyperacute onset (<24 hours)**, copious purulent discharge, lid crusting, preauricular node, papillary reaction	Gram stain: Gram-negative intracellular diplococci Bacterial cultures: On blood + chocolate agar	One dose of **ceftriaxone** (IM) or **ciprofloxacin** (PO) or **ofloxacin** (PO) Ciprofloxacin ophthalmic drops, one drop every 2 hours	Follow up every 2–3 days; ophthalmology evaluation; inquire about other STDs; test and treat all patients for possible *Chlamydia* coinfection
Parinaud oculoglandular syndrome	Mucopurulent discharge, foreign body sensation, granulomatous nodules on palpebral conjunctiva, swollen preauricular or submandibular nodes ipsilaterally, recent contact with a cat or kitten	No routine tests If diagnosis in doubt: Conjunctival biopsy with scrapings (Gram, Giemsa, acid-fast stains), culture (blood, Lowenstein-Jensen, Sabouraud, thioglycolate) Also consider: RPR, FTA-ABS, CXR, tuberculin skin test, blood culture, and cat-scratch serologies	Warm compresses, antipyretics Cat-scratch: Typically self-limited but consider tetracycline, TMP/SMX, or ciprofloxacin for 4 weeks Topical antibiotic bacitracin or polymyxin B ointment four times daily	Laboratory studies not routinely required, but are indicated if no history of recent cat contact (see also tularemia in Biowarfare, Chapter 20)

*All specimens are from conjunctiva unless otherwise noted

Abbreviations: CXR, chest x-ray; ELISA, enzyme-linked immunosorbent assay; FTA-ABS, fluorescent treponemal antibody absorption test; HSV, herpes simplex virus; RPR, rapid plasma reagin; STD, sexually transmitted disease; TMP/SMX, trimethoprim/sulfamethoxazole

■ **Complications**
- Corneal ulcers or infiltrates, preseptal cellulitis, epidemic infectious spread

Infectious Keratitis

Sight-threatening, usually **painful, corneal opacity** or staining

■ **Epidemiology**
- Bacterial: Leading cause of corneal blindness in developing countries. In the US, 10–30 cases per 100,000; 19% to 42% are **contact lens-associated** (less with daily wear soft lenses than with extended wear lenses). Endogenous suppurative keratitis from blood-borne infections is extremely rare
- Viral: 0.15% of US population develop HSV ocular involvement
- Fungal: 5% to 10% of all keratitis in US; increased risk with trauma from organic material or topical steroid use
- Other: *Acanthamoeba* is a higher risk in contact lens wearers who have exposure to fresh water sources

■ **Risk Factors**
- Contact lens wear, especially if worn overnight or with poor lens care
- Trauma, ocular surgery (including LASIK), contaminated ocular medications, immune compromise, dry eye, exposure (remember to tape patients' eyes closed during all surgeries), other ocular surface disease, prior or concurrent herpes infection, corneal graft, topical steroid use

■ **Etiology**
- Common bacterial: *S. aureus, Streptococcus* spp, *P. aeruginosa, Corynebacterium* spp, *Moraxella* spp, *Serratia marcescens, H. influenzae*
- Other bacterial: *N. gonorrhoeae, N. meningitidis, C. trachomatis*
- Common viral: HSV, varicella, adenovirus (serotypes 8 + 19)
- Fungal: *Candida* spp, *Fusarium* spp, *Aspergillus* spp
- Other: *Acanthamoeba, Microsporidium* spp, *Treponema pallidum, Borrelia burgdorferi, Mycobacterium tuberculosis, Mycobacterium leprae,* onchocerciasis, trypanosomiasis

■ **Pathogenesis**
- Corneal epithelial compromise allows infection of corneal epithelium or invasion of stroma
- May lead to ulceration, stromal necrosis, perforation or scarring

■ **History/Physical Exam and Additional Studies** (Table 6-2)

- Obtain ocular and immune status history
- **Document visual acuity** and pupillary exam
- Perform full ophthalmologic exam with **fluorescein staining** and measurement of abnormality
- **Danger signs:** Large central ulcer, severe opacification or visual loss, marked corneal thinning or anterior bulge, corneal perforation (diagnosed by positive Seidel test, which involves painting the eye with fluorescein and observing for leakage), dendritiform lesions, **Hutchinson's sign** (Table 6-2), and marked photophobia

■ **Differential Diagnosis**

- Corneal abrasion, old scar, *Staphylococcus* hypersensitivity, "epidemic keratoconjunctivitis," interstitial keratitis (e.g., syphilis, Lyme, leprosy), keratopathy (Thygeson's, band, filamentary, neurotrophic, bullous), vitamin A deficiency, sterile foreign body or rust ring, exposure, trauma, chemical burn, pterygium, phlyctenule (pink nodule in center of hyperemic conjuctiva, a hypersensitivity reaction), acute angle closure glaucoma, collagen vascular disease, uveitis, endopthalmitis, neoplasm, corneal dystrophy, drug toxicity

■ **Management** (see Table 6-2)

- **Ophthalmology consult:** Unless significant delay is expected, defer antibiotics until ophthalmologic exam and cultures are complete
- No contact lens use or topical steroids until cleared by an ophthalmologist
- **Cycloplegia:** Scopolamine 0.25% or atropine 1% three times daily
- **Oral analgesics** (e.g., acetaminophen ± codeine) as needed
- Consider hospital admission if (1) patient unable to take medication reliably, (2) very severe central ulcers

■ **Complications**

- Vision loss, corneal scarring, opacification, vascularization, perforation, endophthalmitis, iritis. May require long-term therapy and possibly corneal graft

Infectious Endophthalmitis

Sight-threatening **intraocular infection** requiring immediate ophthalmology consult

■ TABLE 6-2   Infectious Keratitis

Organism	Ocular Signs/Symptoms	Evaluation	Treatment	Other
Bacterial	Injected conjunctiva, pain, photophobia, mucus discharge, decreased vision, focal corneal opacity with fluorescein staining	Corneal scrapings for Gram and Giemsa stain and culture (blood, chocolate, Sabaraud, and thioglycolate) Consider corneal biopsy	Generally: Topical polymyxin B/bacitracin or fluoroquinolones* (ciprofloxacin, ofloxacin) every 2–6 hours Severe: Fortified cefazolin and tobramycin alternating every half hour Contact lens wearer: Ciprofloxacin or ofloxacin drops every hour around the clock	Adjust antibiotics based on culture *P. aeruginosa* can rapidly progress to corneal perforation Consider loading doses of antibiotic drops: One drop every 5 minutes three times, then every 15 minutes 12 times, then every hour
Atypical mycobacteria	Typically follows injury or corneal transplants	Acid-fast stain Culture on Lowenstein-Jensen medium (takes ~8 weeks to grow)	Amikacin (10 mg/mL) one drop every 2 hours for 7 days, then four times daily for 2 months	Alternative treatments: Kanamycin or cefoxitin

(Continued)

TABLE 6-2 Continued

Organism	Ocular Signs/Symptoms	Evaluation	Treatment	Other
Fungal	Fluffy **stromal infiltrate** with feathery borders, corneal or stromal epithelial defect, satellite lesions, anterior chamber reaction or hypopyon	Giemsa stain Corneal biopsy	**Natamycin** 5% one drop every 1–2 hours **Cycloplegia** (scopolamine 0.25% three times daily) Severe infection requires amphotericin B, miconazole or clotrimazole drops, or itraconazole PO	Often follows plant-related trauma **Avoid topical steroids** Eye shield, no eye patching. Monitor IOP Corneal transplant for progressive infection or perforation
HSV	Causes epithelial or stromal involvement or anterior uveitis (iritis, corneal scars, iris atrophy) Also may cause diminished corneal sensation and elevated IOP	Rose bengal staining of dendrites on exam Corneal scraping for Giemsa (multinucleated giant cells) or Pap stain (internuclear eosinophilic inclusions), ELISA, and viral culture	Epithelial: **Trifluridine** 1% (Viroptic), one drop nine times daily **Cycloplegia:** Scopolamine (0.25% three times daily), consider debriding dendrites Stromal or uveitis: As above, plus prednisolone acetate 1% four times daily and acyclovir Treat 7–14 days or until resolution	May recur **AVOID topical steroid** with any epithelial defect Monitor IOP

TABLE 6-2 Continued

Organism	Ocular Signs/Symptoms	Evaluation	Treatment	Other
Varicella zoster virus	Vesicular rash in cranial nerve V dermatome, paresthesias, pseudodendrites (raised "stuck-on" mucus plaques) ± elevated IOP; **Hutchinson's sign** (lesions on nose herald ocular involvement)	**Eye findings may precede skin rash** Document date of onset	Cool compresses; bacitracin or erythromycin ophthalmic ointment twice daily Preservative-free artificial tears every 2–6 hours **Prednisolone acetate** 1%, one drop every 1–6 hours **Cycloplegia:** Scopolamine 0.25% three times daily If symptoms present <72 hours, then oral antiviral (acyclovir, valacyclovir) for 7–10 days	Exclude **systemic immune compromise** in patients <40 years If severe with systemic symptoms, consider IV acyclovir and exclude CNS involvement

* Fourth-generation fluoroquinolones (gatifloxacin, levofloxacin, moxifloxacin) are excellent alternatives with better gram-positive coverage, but are not yet FDA approved for corneal ulcer therapy

Abbreviations: CNS, central nervous system; ELISA, enzyme-linked immunorbent assay; HSV, herpes simplex virus; IOP, intraocular pressure

■ Epidemiology/Risk Factors

- **Penetrating ocular trauma:** Up to 30% risk of infection
- Rare complication of ocular surgery (<0.1% of all cataract surgeries) usually presenting within 3–7 days postoperatively
- Glaucoma surgery with filtering bleb carries increased risk of infection for life of bleb (1% to 18% incidence)
- Endogenous etiology rare. Predisposing conditions include immunocompromise (e.g., diabetes, malignancy) and IV drug use

■ Etiology

- Trauma: *Staphylococcus epidermidis*, gram-negative aerobes and anaerobes, *Streptococcus* spp, fungi
- Postoperative: 2–7 days postoperative: **S. epidermidis,** *S. aureus,* viridans group streptococci, *Proteus* spp, *P. aeruginosa*, *H. influenzae*. If >3 weeks, consider *Propionibacterium acnes*
- Endogenous (hematogenous seeding):
  - Fungal: **Candida** spp, *Aspergillus* spp, *Fusarium* spp, *Cryptococcus neoformans*
  - Bacterial: *S. aureus*, *Klebsiella* spp (especially diabetic patients), *Bacillus cereus* (especially IV drug users), *Streptococcus* spp

■ Pathogenesis

- Intraocular injection of bacteria during surgery or following trauma but also possible following chorioretinal seeding of endogenous infections (i.e., endocarditis, gastrointestinal/skin/joint infections)

■ History/Physical Exam

- Obtain ocular and immune status history. **Document visual acuity** and pupillary exam
- Symptoms: Decreased vision, pain, **photophobia**
- Signs: Conjunctival injection, **hypopyon,** cell and flare, iritis, vitritis, chorioretinitis, blebitis, foreign body
- **Danger signs:** Fulminant course, severe vitreous opacification, visual loss

■ Additional Studies

- **Anterior chamber or vitreous biopsy** for Gram stain and cultures
- Consider orbital CT and ultrasound if foreign body suspected (avoid MRI unless metallic foreign body excluded)
- Systemic infection workup if no history of eye surgery or trauma

■ Differential Diagnosis

- Postoperative inflammation, **phacoanaphylaxis** (granulomatous reaction to lens protein following lens rupture), uveitis (sarcoid, pars planitis, Vogt-Koyanagi-Harada syndrome, Lyme), toxoplasmosis, toxocariasis, acute retinal necrosis, cytomegalovirus (CMV), ocular histoplasmosis, syphilis, sympathetic ophthalmia, uveitic-glaucoma-hyphema syndrome, blebitis, intraocular foreign body (especially copper or iron), infectious keratitis, cataract, neoplasm

■ Management

- **Emergent ophthalmology consult:** Unless significant delay expected, postpone antibiotics until eye cultures have been obtained
- Trauma: May require IV antibiotics (vancomycin + either ciprofloxacin or ceftazidime). Remember to **shield the eye** until ophthalmology examines the patient
- Postoperative: Anterior chamber or vitreous biopsy, **intravitreal or subconjunctival antibiotics** (vancomycin + either amikacin or ceftazidime) ± intravitreal steroids, fortified topical antibiotics, if visual acuity worse than ability to detect hand motion then **consider vitrectomy.** Cases with rapid deterioration of vision may require intravenous antibiotics (vancomycin, amikacin ± ceftazidime)
- Endogenous: IV antibiotics vary depending on etiology. Consider empiric fluoroquinolone or ticarcillin-clavulanate or ampicillin-sulbactam

■ Complications

- Severe vision loss (generally, poor vision on presentation means poor visual prognosis), enucleation, cataract, retinal or corneal scarring, opacification, vascularization, perforation, endophthalmitis, iritis. May require long-term therapy and possible corneal graft

Extraocular/Orbital Infection

- Infection of the periocular tissues within the orbit typically caused by local trauma or extension of infection from another area. Potentially life threatening. A variety of presentations and etiologies are possible
- Preseptal cellulitis: Infection of the eyelid anterior to orbital septum; also referred to as periorbital cellulitis
- Orbital cellulitis: Infection posterior to orbital septum
- Dacryocystitis: Infection of the nasolacrimal sac

■ Epidemiology/Risk Factors

- Preseptal cellulitis: **Local trauma** is the major risk factor

- Orbital cellulitis: 90% are secondary to **extension of bacterial sinusitis.** Other risk factors include dental infections, facial trauma, endophthalmitis, septic embolization
- Dacryocystitis: Associated with nasolacrimal duct obstruction

■ Etiology/Pathogenesis

- Preseptal: *S. aureus*, *Streptococcus* spp, *Haemophilus influenzae*, HSV, VZV ± bacterial superinfection
- Orbital: *S. aureus*, *Streptococcus* spp, gram-negative rods, anaerobes, *Mucor*, *Aspergillus*
- Dacryocystitis: *S. aureus*, *Streptococcus* spp, diphtheroids

■ History/Physical Exam (Table 6-3)

- Ocular and immune status history, vision, pupillary exam, exophthalmometry
- **Danger signs:** Sudden onset, vision loss, limited and painful eye movements, fluctuant mass, proptosis

■ Differential Diagnosis

- Thyroid eye disease, orbital pseudotumor, trauma, neoplasm (primary or metastatic), arteriovenous fistula (carotid cavernous fistula), orbital varix, vasculitis (i.e., Wegener's), optic neuritis, mucocele, dermoid, hemangioma, lymphangioma, meningioma, sarcoid, neurofibromatosis, tuberous sclerosis, cranial nerve palsy, shallow orbits, contralateral enophthalmos or ptosis, conjunctivitis, insect bite

■ Management (see Table 6-3)

■ Complications

- Septic cavernous sinus thrombosis, intracranial abscess, vision loss, death, orbital apex syndrome

■ TABLE 6-3 Orbital Infection

Infection	Ocular Signs/Symptoms	Evaluation	Treatment	Other
Preseptal cellulitis	Tender, warm, erythematous lid edema, ± mild fever, chemosis	Gram stain and culture any wound Orbital CT if limited or painful extraocular movements or photophobia	Warm compress Polymyxin B/bacitracin ointment four times daily Afebrile, reliable patient with mild case: Amoxicillin-clavulanate, cefaclor, or TMP/SMX Moderate-severe, or unreliable patient, or refractive to oral therapy: Ceftriaxone and vancomycin Total antibiotic duration: 10–14 days	Bacteremia less common in post-*Haemophilus influenzae* type b era
Orbital cellulitis	Same as preseptal but with **pain on eye movements**, fever, decreased vision, headache, diplopia, **proptosis** or globe displacement, retinal venous congestion, optic disk edema, purulent discharge, ± sinusitis	**Contrast CT or MRI** of orbits/sinuses ± brain, CBC (WBC usually elevated), blood culture, evaluation for meningitis ENT consult for evaluation and possible sinus drainage	**Ceftriaxone and vancomycin** (add metronidazole if at risk for anaerobic infection), or ampicillin–sulbactam Nasal decongestant (e.g., Afrin twice daily), no nose blowing Total antibiotic duration: 14–21 days (large undrained collections may require longer treatment)	May require exploration or incisional drainage; watch for subperiosteal abscess; risk of septic **cavernous sinus thrombosis**; if immune-compromised or diabetic, consider mucormycosis (biopsy necrotic site)

(Continued)

■ TABLE 6-3 Continued

Infection	Ocular Signs/Symptoms	Evaluation	Treatment	Other
Dacryocystitis	Tearing; discharge; raised, inflamed nodular lesion just inferior to the medial canthus (lacrimal sac); ±fistula formation	**Mucoid discharge may be expressed from punctum** for Gram stain and culture Consider CT if severe or refractory to therapy	Warm compress/massage of nasolacrimal duct Trimethoprim/polymyxin one drop four times daily Afebrile, reliable patient with mild case: Cephalexin or amoxicillin-clavulanate Moderate-severe, febrile, unreliable patient, or refractive to oral therapy: **Cefazolin** Total antibiotic duration: 10–14 days	Consider incisional drainage of nasolacrimal duct if pointing abscess; may need surgical correction (dacryocystorhinostomy) if chronic or recurrent

Abbreviations: CBC, complete blood count; CT, computed tomography; ENT, ear, nose, and throat; MRI, magnetic resonance imaging; TMP/SMX, trimethoprim-sulfamethoxazole; WBC, white blood cell

Central Nervous System Infections

Lee S. Engel, MD, PhD and Fred A. Lopez, MD

Meningitis

Categories include bacterial meningitis, viral meningitis (aseptic meningitis), and chronic meningitis
- **Bacterial meningitis** is relatively more common in **winter**
- **Viral meningitis** is more common in **summer**

■ Epidemiology

- 4% of population will develop either bacterial or viral meningitis before the age of 80
- The overall **mortality rate** for bacterial meningitis is **10%**

■ Risk Factors

- Age over 60 or under 5 years
- Acute and chronic otitis media; sinusitis; pneumonia; **endocarditis**; head injury; recent neurosurgery; cerebrospinal fluid (CSF) shunts; CSF leak; diabetes mellitus; alcoholism; altered immune status; IV drug use; recent exposure to others with meningitis; sickle cell disease; crowding (**military and college dorms**)
- Asplenia: Increased risk of infection with encapsulated organisms (*Streptococcus pneumoniae*, *Neisseria meningitidis*, *Haemophilus influenzae*)
- **Terminal (C5–C9) complement deficiencies**: Increased risk of infection with *N. meningitidis*

■ Etiology

- Bacterial meningitis (Table 7-1)
- Viral meningitis
  - Enteroviruses (coxsackievirus, echovirus, and poliovirus) cause more than half the cases of acute viral meningitis
  - Herpes simplex virus 1 (HSV-1); HSV-2; varicella-zoster virus (VZV); HIV
- Chronic meningitis
  - *Mycobacterium*, *Cryptococcus*, *Coccidioides*, *Blastomyces*, *Histoplasma*, *Sporothrix*, syphilis, Lyme disease, leptospirosis, *Toxoplasma*, *Acanthamoeba*

■ TABLE 7-1 Pathogens in Community-Acquired Bacterial Meningitis				
Age < 1 Month	Age 1–23 Months	Age 2–18 Years	Age 19–59 Years	Age > 60 Years
Group B streptococci	S. pneumoniae	N. meningitidis	S. pneumoniae	S. pneumoniae
Listeria monocytogenes	N. meningitidis	S. pneumoniae	N. meningitidis	Listeria monocytogenes
E. coli	Group B streptococci	H. influenzae	H. influenzae	H. influenzae

■ Pathogenesis

- Bacterial meningitis: Initial colonization of mucosal surfaces, including the nasopharynx, followed by either hematogenous spread to the central nervous system (CNS) or contiguous spread from a cranial site of infection
- Viral meningitis: Infection of the mucosal surfaces of the respiratory tract or gastrointestinal tract followed by viremia with hematogenous spread to the CNS

■ History

- Classic symptoms include **fever, headache, and stiff neck**
- Chills, **photophobia**, nausea and vomiting, seizures, altered sensorium, and focal neurological symptoms
- May have antecedent upper respiratory tract infection
- Bacterial meningitis is more sudden in onset than viral meningitis

■ Physical Exam

- **Nuchal rigidity** or discomfort with neck flexion
- Jolt test: Headache worsens when the patient's head is turned horizontally at a frequency of two or three rotations per second
- **Kernig's sign:** Resistance or pain in the lower back or thigh when extending the knee of the patient lying supine with the **hip flexed at 90°**
- **Brudzinski's sign: Passive neck flexion** causes the supine patient to actively flex the hips and knees
- Neurological findings include altered mental status, cranial nerve dysfunction (III, VI, and VIII most common), seizures, hemiparesis, visual field defects, papilledema, or aphasia
- Meningococcal meningitis may present with a rash on the extremities that is initially macular but rapidly evolves into petechiae and then **purpura**

▮ TABLE 7-2   CSF Findings in Various Forms of Meningitis

	Opening Pressure (mm H$_2$0)	WBC[a]	Glucose (mg/dL)	Protein (mg/dL)	Organisms in the CSF
Normal values	90–180	0–5 lymphocytes	50–75	15–40	None
Bacterial meningitis	>180	1000–5000 PMNs	<40	100–500	Gram stain positive 60% to 90% Culture positive 70% to 85%
Viral meningitis	90–200	10–300; may see up to 80% PMNs in early infection	Normal	50–100	Gram stain negative Some viruses recoverable such as HSV-2 and enteroviruses
Cryptococcal meningitis	180–300	10–200 lymphocytes	<40	50–200	India ink positive 25% to 50% Culture and antigen positive > 90%
Tuberculosis meningitis	180–300	<500 lymphocytes	<50	100–200	AFB smear positive 10% to 22% AFB culture positive 38% to 88%
Lyme meningitis	90–200	10–300 lymphocytes	Normal	50–100	None

Abbreviations: AFB, acid-fast bacilli; PMN, polymorphonuclear cell

■ Additional Studies

• Lumbar puncture with opening pressure measurement (Table 7-2)
  - CSF tube #1 for glucose and protein
  - CSF tube #2 for cell count and differential
  - CSF tube #3 for bacterial and fungal culture, Gram stain, India ink, acid-fast bacilli (AFB) cultures, VDRL, and cryptococcal antigen
  - CSF tube #4 for viral studies and cytology
• Complete blood count, chemistry panel; cultures of blood, urine, and sputum; chest x-ray; serology for syphilis and Lyme disease; purified protein derivative (PPD); electroencephalogram (EEG)
• Computed tomography (CT) scan of the head before lumbar puncture may be indicated for patients older than 60, immunocompromised, have a history of central nervous system disease,

had a seizure within 1 week before presentation, or have neurological deficits

■ Differential Diagnosis

- Brain abscess, intracranial tumor or hemorrhage, cysticercosis, hypersensitivity to drugs (e.g., sulfonamides, nonsteroidal anti-inflammatory drugs [NSAIDs]), systemic lupus erythematosus (SLE), Behçet's syndrome, sarcoidosis

■ Management

- Empiric management of bacterial meningitis (Table 7-3)
- **Dexamethasone** has been shown to improve outcome and reduce mortality associated with pneumococcal meningitis when given before or during antibiotic administration
- Prevention of Meningococcal meningitis for high-risk people (dormitory, military) with meningococcal vaccine
- **Prophylaxis** for contacts of people with Meningococcal meningitis with **rifampin, ciprofloxacin, or ceftriaxone**

■ Complications

- Seizures, elevated intracranial pressure, cerebral thrombosis, hydrocephalus, ataxia, blindness, deafness, death

Encephalitis

- Acute viral encephalitis results from direct infection of the neural cells, resulting in neuronal destruction and tissue necrosis (i.e., affects the gray matter)
- Postinfectious encephalomyelitis follows a variety of viral and bacterial infections, causing widespread periventricular inflammation and demyelination without direct infection of the neuronal cells (i.e., affects the white matter)
- Vast number of causative organisms, and only few are treatable

■ Epidemiology

- 20,000 cases of encephalitis in the US each year
- Epidemiological factors such as season, work exposure, history of tick bite, residence in or travel to endemic areas will help differentiate the possible causes

■ Risk Factors

- Age: Neonates and adults older than 60
- Epidemiologic factors

■ Etiology (Table 7-4)

- In the US, the most common cause is HSV-1

■ TABLE 7-3   Initial Antibiotic Therapy for Community-Acquired Bacterial Meningitis

Age or Condition	Likely Pathogen	Empiric Antibiotic
0–4 weeks	Group B streptococci *Escherichia coli* *L. monocytogenes*	Ampicillin + cefotaxime or ampicillin + aminoglycoside
4–12 weeks	Group B streptococci *E. coli* *L. monocytogenes* *H. influenzae* *S. pneumoniae*	Ampicilin + either cefotaxime or ceftriaxone
3 months to 17 years	*S. pneumoniae* *N. meningitidis* *H. influenzae*	Vancomycin + 3rd generation cephalosporin (i.e., cefotaxime or ceftriaxone)
18–50 years	*S. pneumoniae* *N. meningitidis*	Vancomycin + 3rd generation cephalosporin (i.e., cefotaxime or ceftriaxone) Penicillin-allergic: Chloramphenicol + trimethoprim/sulfamethoxazole + vancomycin
>50 years	*S. pneumoniae* *N. meningitidis* *L. monocytogenes*	Cefotaxime or ceftriaxone + vancomycin + ampicillin **Penicillin-allergic:** Vancomycin + trimethoprim/sulfamethoxazole
Impaired cellular immunity	*L. monocytogenes* Gram-negative bacteria *Staphylococcus aureus*	Ampicillin + ceftazidime + vancomycin
Basilar skull fracture or CSF leak	*S. pneumoniae* Various streptococci *H. influenzae* *N. meningitidis*	Vancomycin + 3rd generation cephalosporin (i.e., cefotaxime or ceftriaxone)
CSF mechanical shunt	*S. aureus* Coagulase-negative staphylococci *Pseudomonas aeruginosa* Enterobacteriaceae	Vancomycin + ceftazidime

■ TABLE 7-4   Causes of Encephalitis

Seasonal	Nonseasonal
Viral-mosquito borne	**Viral**
La Crosse (California group)	HSV-1
St. Louis	HSV-2
Western equine	VZV
Eastern equine	Epstein-Barr virus
Japanese	Human herpesvirus 6
Venezuelan	Adenovirus
West Nile virus	Enterovirus
	Rabies
Viral-tick borne	CMV
Powassan	Poliovirus
Colorado tick	Measles
Bacterial	Mumps
Rocky Mountain spotted fever	**Parasitic**
Ehrlichiosis	Toxoplasmosis
Lyme	
Leptospirosis	
Listeria monocytogenes	
Amoeba	
Naegleria	
Acanthamoeba	

■ Pathogenesis

- Respiratory or person-to-person transmission seen with measles, mumps, enteroviruses, and herpesviruses resulting in viremia
- Inoculation into bloodstream seen with mosquito- and tick-borne viruses

■ History

- Variable onset of febrile illness with prominent headache; altered level of consciousness; behavioral and speech disturbances; focal signs (seizures or paresis)
- Gastrointestinal disturbances with enteroviruses
- Animal exposure (e.g., animal bite for rabies)
- Geographic exposure

■ Physical Exam

- Findings may be associated with specific illnesses (Table 7-5)

■ TABLE 7-5 Clinical Clues to the Causes of Encephalitis

Cause	Clues
Herpes simplex virus	Temporal lobe signs such as personality change and hallucinations; fever almost always present; associated with primary HSV infection in 30% of cases; MRI reveals abnormalities in the temporal lobe
Varicella-zoster virus	Cerebellar ataxia in children and progressive confusion in adults; patients may have a vesiculopustular eruption
Epstein-Barr virus	Meningoencephalitis in adults; patients may have pharyngitis, lymphadenopathy, and splenomegaly
Human herpesvirus 6	Focal encephalitis in adults
Cytomegalovirus	Slowly progressive; may appear like AIDS dementia
Enteroviruses	May occur in epidemics; patients may have a diffuse rash, gastroenteritis, or upper respiratory tract infection
Poliovirus	Involvement of the spinal cord and brainstem
Japanese encephalitis virus	Brainstem involvement; meningeal signs; parkinsonian signs
West Nile virus	Areas where there is the unexpected death of birds; 20% to 30% of patients have decreased muscle strength, erythematous rash, and lymphocytopenia; older age associated with more severe neurological disease
Rabies virus	Hyperesthesia at inoculation (bite) site
Postinfectious encephalomyelitis	Associated with varicella-zoster, measles, mumps, rubella, Epstein-Barr, and influenza viruses; occurs days to weeks after viral symptoms with sudden fever, obtundation, and focal signs; MRI demonstrates multifocal white matter lesions
Toxoplasmosis	Ring-enhancing lesions on CT or MRI
L. monocytogenes	Occurs at extremes of age; frequently produces microabscesses in the brain stem
Rocky Mountain spotted fever	Peak in early summer; high fever; headache and myalgias; a petechial rash forms that becomes purpuric on the wrists, ankles, palms, and soles
Amebic	Swimming in freshwater lakes; usually fatal disease

Abbreviations: AIDS, acquired immune deficiency syndrome; MRI, magnetic resonance imaging; CT, computed tomography

■ Additional Studies

• Lumbar puncture as for meningitis, but also send **CSF for polymerase chain reaction (PCR) to detect HSV, varicella-zoster, Lyme disease, and human herpesvirus 6**; virus-specific IgM antibodies for arboviruses; viral culture for enteroviruses

- Complete blood count (CBC); serum chemistries; coagulation profile; urine electrolytes (if syndrome of inappropriate antidiuretic hormone [SIADH] suspected); serological tests for toxoplasmosis
- MRI, head CT with and without contrast, EEG
- Brain biopsy (which is rarely indicated) for HSV or rabies

■ Differential Diagnosis

- Meningitis, brain abscess, neurosyphilis, ehrlichiosis, metabolic disturbances, thiamine deficiency (Wernicke's encephalopathy), sarcoidosis, cerebral vasculitis, Guillain-Barré syndrome, SLE, Wegener's granulomatosis

■ Management

- High-dose intravenous **acyclovir for HSV**
- Doxycycline if Rocky Mountain spotted fever, ehrlichiosis, or Lyme disease suspected
- Amphotericin B if Naegleria infection suspected

■ Complications

- **Seizures,** increased intracranial pressure, **SIADH,** motor and sensory deficits, coma, death

Brain and Parameningeal Abscesses

- Brain abscess is a focal, intracerebral infection that begins as a local area of cerebritis and develops into a collection of pus
- Brain abscess is uncommon and presents insidiously with few systemic signs of infection

■ Epidemiology

- 1 in 10,000 hospital admissions for brain abscess in the US
- Mortality for persons with brain abscess is about 10%
- Brain abscess is most frequent in people aged 20–40 years

■ Risk Factors

- Male sex, **penetrating head trauma**, ischemia, infarction, contusion, chronic otitis media, mastoiditis, cholesteatomas, dental infections, surgical procedures including resection of nasal septum, placement of cranial traction with a halo, **pulmonary arteriovenous malformations**, carotid endarterectomy, preeclampsia, ventriculostomy, meningitis caused by *Citrobacter diversus* and *L. monocytogenes*, IV drug use

■ Etiology

- Predominant organisms include *Streptococcus milleri*, *Bacteroides* spp, *S. aureus*, *Proteus* spp, and diphtheroids

- In the immunocompromised host, consider *Aspergillus, Candida, Cryptococcus, Nocardia,* and *Toxoplasma*
- Other causes include *Mycobacterium tuberculosis, Entamoeba histolytica,* and neurocysticercosis due to *Taenia solium*

■ Pathogenesis

- The infectious agent can enter the brain through direct spread from a focal cranial infection or trauma
- The infectious agent can enter the brain via hematogenous seeding, often causing multiple abscesses

■ History

- **Headache** characterized by **poorly localized** dull ache that may progress to pain localized to the side of the abscess
- Changes in mental status, lethargy, progressing to coma—associated with poor prognosis
- Vomiting in association with **increased intracranial pressure**

■ Physical Exam

- Fever, focal neurological deficits, seizures, and cranial nerve III and VI defects indicate increased intracranial pressure; papilledema is a late manifestation of cerebral edema

■ Additional Studies

- Lumbar puncture contraindicated in presence of focal neurologic symptoms or papilledema
- CT scan not as sensitive as MRI but may be obtained more easily on an emergent basis
- Diagnostic aspiration with Gram stain, aerobic and anaerobic cultures

■ Differential Diagnosis

- Cerebral aneurysm, septic cerebral emboli, stroke, acute focal necrotizing encephalitis, metastatic or primary brain tumors, pyogenic meningitis, migraine headache, hypertensive emergencies, extradural abscess, sinus thrombosis

■ Management

- Blood cultures should be drawn and empiric antibiotics started before CT or MRI
- **Empiric antibiotic therapy** with a third-generation cephalosporin and metronidazole for most brain abscesses
- Vancomycin, third generation cephalosporin ± metronidazole for brain abscesses caused by penetrating head injury
- Vancomycin for brain abscesses associated with neurosurgical procedures

- **Drainage of abscess larger than 4 cm**
- Corticosteroids have no impact on survival, sequelae, or length of hospital stay, but are useful to decrease cerebral edema and intracranial pressure
- Duration of antibiotics typically **4–6 weeks**
- Repeat CT or MRI to document abscess resolution
- Ring-enhancing lesions may take 3–4 months to resolve

■ Complications
- Focal neurological sequelae are usually minor; seizures, meningiomas, and gliosarcomas may develop in patients previously treated for brain abscesses; uncal or tonsillar herniation; abscess hemorrhage or rupture

Ventricular Shunt Infections

- 95% of CSF shunts drain into either the peritoneal cavity (ventriculoperitoneal [VP] shunts) or the right atrium (ventriculoatrial [VA] shunts)

■ Epidemiology
- The lifetime frequency of shunt infections averages 3% to 10%

■ Risk Factors
- Age, history of previous shunt infection, head trauma, surgical technique, and experience of the neurosurgeon

■ Etiology
- ***Staphylococcus epidermidis* accounts for 36% to 80% of cases**
- *S. aureus* accounts for 25%
- Gram-negative enteric bacteria (with VP shunts) account for 5% to 10%
- Anaerobic skin flora (*Propionibacterium* spp) account for 2% to 35%

■ Pathogenesis
- Organisms directly colonize the shunt at the time of surgery
  - 70% of cases manifest **within 2 months of surgery**
- Organisms reach the CSF and shunt by hematogenous spread
  - Patients with VA shunts may be infected following bacteremia or endocarditis
- Organisms travel in a retrograde fashion from the contaminated distal end of the shunt

■ History
- Progressive deterioration of consciousness

- Acute abdominal symptoms such as fullness, vomiting, and poor appetite
- Shunt infection often presents as shunt malfunction

■ Physical Exam

- Fever (temperature over 100°F [38°C]); signs of inflammation along the course of the shunt catheter, signs of bacteremia or **immune complex nephritis in VA shunts**

■ Additional Studies

- Culture any shunt material removed during revision or replacement
- Check for shunt malfunction: Needle aspiration of shunt, CT of brain and abdomen, contrast radiographic studies of the shunt
- Check for wound or shunt track inflammation: Culture of inflamed area, shunt aspiration of CSF, lumbar puncture (LP)
- For a VA shunt: Blood culture, shunt aspiration of CSF, evaluation for right-sided endocarditis, chest x-ray, sputum culture and Gram stain, serum complement, circulating immune complexes, urine sedimentation rate
- For a VP shunt: Shunt aspiration of CSF, aspiration of inflammation along distal catheter, evaluation of surgical abdomen

■ Differential Diagnosis

- Shunt obstruction or disconnection, pseudocyst, subdural hematoma

■ Management

- Standard treatment of shunt infections includes complete replacement of the shunt system and intensive antibiotic therapy
- Treat empirically with **vancomycin and ceftazidime** or vancomycin and rifampin; add an aminoglycoside if culture demonstrates gram-negative bacteria (*Pseudomonas* or a coliform)
- Intraventricular vancomycin or nafcillin should be administered along with systemic antibiotics if staphylococci are present
- Antibiotic prophylaxis with vancomycin or a beta-lactam antibiotic for patients with VA shunts who are facing dental or other procedures that can cause bacteremia

■ Complications

- Meningitis; bacteremia; peritonitis; obstruction or perforation can occur with VP shunts; decreased cognitive function in infants who have had shunt infections

Chapter

8 Ear, Nose, and Throat Infections

Greg E. Davis, MD, MPH

Otitis

- **Acute otitis externa** (AOE): Infection of the skin of the external auditory canal
- **Acute otitis media** (AOM): Infection of the middle ear space for less than 3 weeks
- **Otitis media with effusion** (OME): Fluid in the middle ear without active infection
- **Chronic otitis media** (COM): Infection of the middle ear for more than 6 weeks
- **Chronic suppurative otitis media** (CSOM): Chronic tympanomastoiditis with tympanic membrane perforation

■ Epidemiology

- AOM: Second most common disease in children, and the **leading cause of hearing loss** in children

■ Risk Factors

- AOE: Immunocompromised patients, swimmers, children
- AOM: Young age (tortuous eustachian tube), nasopharyngeal mass in adults
- OME: Bottle feeding (rather than breast feeding), passive smoke, group childcare

■ Etiology

- Organisms for AOE: *Pseudomonas aeruginosa*, *Staphylococcus aureus*, other gram-negatives, *Candida albicans*
- AOM: *Streptococcus pneumoniae*, *Haemophilus influenzae*, *Moraxella catarrhalis*, also viral pathogens
- OME: No pathogens present
- COM/CSOM: *P. aeruginosa*, *S. aureus*, and anaerobes

■ Pathogenesis

- AOE: **Microtrauma** (cotton swabs) or **water retention** (swimmers, impacted cerumen)

64

- AOM: **Eustachian tube dysfunction** leads to negative pressure in the middle ear with transudation of fluid followed by inoculation by pathogens
- OME: Chronic **eustachian tube dysfunction**
- COM/CSOM: **Inadequate treatment of AOM**

■ History

- AOE: Pruritus, otalgia, otorrhea, conductive hearing loss
- AOM: Otalgia, aural fullness, fever, irritability
- CSOM: Painful ear with otorrhea

■ Physical Exam

- AOE: Edema, erythema, squamous debris, and tenderness of the external auditory canal and tragus
- AOM: Hyperemic tympanic membrane, middle ear effusion. On pneumatic otoscopy, **nonmobile tympanic membrane (TM)**, **air-fluid level**
- OME: **Effusion** in the middle ear space on pneumatic otoscopy with no signs of inflammation
- CSOM: **Purulent** otorrhea with TM perforation

■ Additional Studies

- AOE: None
- AOM: Tympanometry is useful when the TM cannot be clearly visualized. Normal tympanometry excludes the diagnosis of AOM
- OME: **Hearing evaluation** (audiogram) after 3 months of documented effusion or if any language delay, learning problems, or a significant hearing loss is suspected

■ Differential Diagnosis

- Important note: In unilateral AOM in adults, **nasopharyngeal disease** (such as nasopharyngeal carcinoma) should be considered
- Referred pain from teeth or jaw, cavernous sinus thrombosis

■ Management

- AOE:
  - Dry ear precautions
  - Apply otic drops (neomycin/polymyxin/hydrocortisone [Cortisporin or CiproDex])
  - Oral antibiotics are not necessary

- AOM:
  - 50% of cases resolve spontaneously, oral coverage for most likely pathogens for 10 days (amoxicillin). If no improvement within 3 days, broaden coverage (amoxicillin-clavulanate, levofloxacin). Also consider analgesics, antipyretics, and nasal decongestants
- Tympanocentesis reserved for very rare situations of significant immunocompromised status where a culture is necessary for effective treatment, or in the neonatal patient unresponsive to appropriate therapy.
- OME:
  - Hearing evaluation if fluid present for more than 3 months, and consider bilateral myringotomy and pressure equalization tube (BMT) placement if hearing loss
- COM:
  - Consider BMT with or without adenoidectomy
- CSOM:
  - Ofloxacin or ciprofloxacin suspension ear drops with oral coverage as above

■ Complications

- AOE: External auditory canal stenosis, malignant otitis externa (necrotizing infection that spreads from squamous epithelium of ear canal to adjacent areas of soft tissue and bone; more common in those with diabetes)
- AOM/COM: Tympanic membrane perforation, tympanosclerosis, cholesteatoma, hearing loss (with subsequent speech delay), mastoiditis (1 in 400 with AOM), epidural/subdural/brain abscesses, meningitis

Sinusitis (Rhinosinusitis)

- Acute bacterial rhinosinusitis (ABR): Symptoms present for at least 10 days, but less than 28 days
- Subacute rhinosinusitis: 28 days to 12 consecutive weeks
- Chronic rhinosinusitis (CRS): More than 12 consecutive weeks of symptoms. Must also classify presence or absence of nasal polyps.

■ Epidemiology

- Chronic sinusitis is the most common self-reported chronic condition in the US
- 33 million cases each year in the US

- **Risk factors:** Allergy, maxillofacial trauma, immunodeficiency, noxious chemicals/pollutants, surgery, mucociliary dysfunction, nasal polyposis

Etiology

- ABR: *S. pneumoniae, H. influenzae,* and *M. catarrhalis*
- CRS: Same as ABR plus *S. aureus* and anaerobes

Pathogenesis

- ABR is usually **preceded by a viral URI,** which can lead to inflammation of the paranasal sinus mucosa, obstruction of the natural drainage pathways, and pathogenic bacterial superinfection
- CRS is usually secondary to persistent obstruction of natural drainage pathways or nasal polyposis.

History

- ABR can be diagnosed after 10 days of viral URI symptoms or after 5 days of worsening symptoms
- **Symptoms:** Facial pain or pressure, nasal congestion, rhinorrhea, postnasal drip, fever, cough, myalgia, hyposmia/anosmia, maxillary dental pain, or ear pressure/fullness
- Note: Color of nasal drainage is not an indicator for bacterial versus viral rhinosinusitis

Physical Exam

- Facial pain with manual pressure on the paranasal sinuses
- Anterior rhinoscopy: Purulent drainage in the anterior nasal cavity
- Nasal endoscopy: Purulence in the middle meatus

Additional Studies

- CT scan is the radiologic method of choice, but is indicated only during surgical decision-making and is not necessary for routine diagnosis

Differential Diagnosis

- Migraines, allergic rhinitis, temporomandibular joint disorder, myofacial pain, dental abscess, nasopharyngeal neoplasm

Management

- ABR: Oral coverage 10 days with amoxicillin with or without clavulanate, or erythromycin plus trimethoprim-sulfamethoxazole (TMP/SMX) for penicillin allergies, or cefpodoxime proxetil, cefuroxime axetil, or cefdinir if no recent use of antibiotics (in previous 4–6 weeks). If recent antibiotic use or if severe

disease, then fluoroquinolone or high-dose amoxicillin/clavulanate. Also analgesics, antipyretics, and nasal decongestants. Failure to improve within 72 hours of antibiotics should prompt reevaluation and alternative antimicrobial agent
• CRS: Amoxicillin/clavulanate, fluoroquinolone or cefuroxime. Recommended duration is 21 days

■ Complications
• Meningitis, subdural/epidural abscess, orbital cellulitis, subperiorbital abscess, cavernous sinus thrombosis

Pharyngitis

■ Epidemiology
• Inflammation of the mucosal and submucosal structures of the throat
• Accounts for 15% of all office visits
• Peak seasons are winter and spring
• Group A beta-hemolytic streptococcus (GABHS) cause 5% to 10% of episodes in adults and 15% to 30% in children

■ Risk Factors
• Young age
• Daycare or community living
• Diabetes or immunocompromise

■ Etiology
• Usually viral (rhinovirus, adenovirus, and enterovirus). Secondary bacterial infections are caused by GABHS (*Streptococcus pyogenes*), *S. pneumoniae, H. influenzae*
• Other causes of chronic pharyngitis: Gastroesophageal reflux disease (GERD), neoplasm (squamous cell carcinoma, lymphoma), postnasal drip, smoking
• Uncommon causes: Syphilis, *Neisseria gonorrhoeae, Mycoplasma pneumoniae, Chlamydophila pneumoniae*, pertussis, candidiasis, infectious mononucleosis, herpangina, diphtheria, and scarlet fever

■ Pathogenesis
• Symptoms develop 1–3 days after exposure

■ History/Physical Exam
• Sore throat, odynophagia, malaise, fever, referred otalgia
• Concurrent rhinorrhea or cough suggests viral pharyngitis

- Features suggesting **viral etiology** include
  - Conjunctivitis, cough, coryza, diarrhea
  - Discrete ulcerative lesions
  - Hoarse voice (laryngitis)
- Features suggestive of GABHS include
  - Tonsillar swelling
  - Tender, enlarged anterior cervical nodes
  - Scarlatiniform rash
  - Exposure to person with GABHS pharyngitis

■ Additional Studies

- **Throat cultures:** Rapid streptococcal antigen test ("rapid strep" test) or standard culture if sore throat persists more than 7 days, and Monospot (blood test) to test for mononucleosis
- Most GABHS **rapid antigen tests** have specificity of 95% or greater, and sensitivity of 80% to 90% (false positives unusual but false negatives may occur)

■ Differential Diagnosis

- Viral or bacterial pharyngitis, herpangina, neoplasm, mononucleosis

■ Management

- Supportive care: Antipyretics, saline gargle rinse, hydration, anesthetic lozenges or sprays
- Antibiotics if rapid strep test is positive (amoxicillin or clindamycin for 10 days or intramuscular benzathine penicillin G, one dose). Second-line antibiotic choices include first- (e.g., cephalexin) or second-generation (e.g., cefuroxime) cephalosporins or macrolides (clarithromycin, azithromycin)
- Except under special circumstances, repeat testing of asymptomatic patients following treatment or routine testing of asymptomatic household contacts is not necessary

■ Complications

- Peritonsillar abscess, retropharyngeal abscess, sepsis
- Tonsillar hypertrophy and associated obstructive sleep disturbance or other airway obstruction
- If GABHS: Poststreptococcal glomerulonephritis, scarlet fever, or rheumatic fever

Respiratory Tract Infections

Chris Knight, MD and Douglas Paauw, MD

Bronchitis

- **Acute bronchitis** is caused by inflammation of the bronchi. The cardinal clinical symptom is cough
- **Chronic bronchitis** is defined as a cough productive of copious sputum for at least 3 months a year for at least 2 consecutive years

■ Epidemiology

- Most acute bronchitis is **due to viral infections,** occurring more commonly in the winter months
- The majority of patients with chronic bronchitis smoke cigarettes

■ Etiology

- Viruses cause almost all acute bronchitis (rhinovirus, respiratory syncytial virus [RSV], influenza, parainfluenza)
- Pertussis is likely the most common bacterial cause of acute bronchitis in patients with coughs lasting more than 2 weeks
- Mycoplasma pneumonia and chlamydia pneumonia make up less than 5% of acute bronchitis in young adults

■ Pathophysiology

Acute Bronchitis

- Variable inflammation of bronchi with little damage caused by rhinovirus, and extensive epithelial damage and destruction caused by influenza. Tracheal and bronchial edema and mucus production lead to bronchospasm and cough

Chronic Bronchitis

- Increased number of mucus-producing goblet cells replace normal ciliated epithelial cells in the bronchial epithelium. Mucus production and hypertrophy of mucosal glands lead to airway narrowing. Infection with bacteria can add to the inflammation and obstruction

■ History/Physical Exam

- **Cough** is the major symptom of bronchitis

Acute Bronchitis

- Associated rhinorrhea is common. The cough is dry and non-productive at the start. May produce small amounts of sputum later in the course. **Fever is not present.** Occasional wheeze may occur

Chronic Bronchitis

- Productive cough with increased volume of mucus production, increasing dyspnea and wheezing

■ Additional Studies

- White blood cell (WBC) count and chest x-ray (CXR) are usually normal in patients with acute bronchitis

■ Differential Diagnosis

- Asthma, postnasal drip, gastroesophageal reflux disease (GERD), congestive heart failure (CHF)
- Pollution/smoke inhalation

■ Management

Acute Bronchitis

- Avoidance of irritants (smoke, perfume)
- Cough suppressants with codeine may offer a small benefit
- **No role for antibiotics** in almost all cases. Antibiotics effective for pertussis only if given within first 7 days of symptoms
- Beta-agonist may be beneficial

Chronic Bronchitis

- Avoidance of smoking
- With chronic obstructive pulmonary disease (COPD) exacerbations, and increased sputum production, can use antibiotics: Amoxicillin, doxycycline, or trimethoprim-sulfamethoxazole (TMP-SMX) are first line. With fever, severe symptoms, and lack of response to first-line antibiotics, options include amoxicillin-clavulanate, cefuroxime, levofloxacin, gatifloxacin, moxifloxacin
- Corticosteroids during COPD exacerbation can be helpful

■ Complications

- Prolonged cough after viral bronchitis can occur
- **With pertussis, cough can last 3–4 months**

Pleural Effusions

- Pleural effusion: Fluid between the parietal and visceral pleura
  - **Transudate:** Noninflammatory effusion, usually due to CHF, nephrotic syndrome, cirrhosis

- **Exudate:** High-protein effusions, turbid. Usually due to malignancy, infection, parapneumonic, or pulmonary embolus (pulmonary infarction)
- **Empyema:** Purulent, a complication of bacterial or fungal pneumonia

■ Epidemiology

- About 10% of patients hospitalized on medicine wards have a pleural effusion
- Half of exudative pleural effusions are parapneumonic effusions

■ Risk Factors

- Alcoholism, injection drug use, and central nervous system (CNS) disease that predisposes to aspiration pneumonia

■ Etiology

- Common cause of pneumonia with parapneumonic effusion: *Streptococcus pneumoniae*
- Less common: *Staphylococcus aureus*, tuberculosis, anaerobic infection, mycoplasma pneumonia, viral
- Common causes of empyema: *S. aureus* and anaerobic infection

■ Pathogenesis

- Pleural effusion develops when the amount of pleural fluid that enters the pleural space exceeds the amount removed via lymphatics. Pleural effusions can be due to increased pleural fluid formation, decreased lymphatic clearance, or a combination of both

■ History

- **Pleuritic chest pain,** dyspnea, and cough are common features
- Think of pleural effusion when patients with pneumonia fail to improve or worsen on antibiotics

■ Physical Exam

- Dullness to percussion, decreased breath sounds, and decreased tactile fremitus

■ Additional Studies

- CXR: **Costophrenic angle blunting** (need 175 mL to see costophrenic angle blunting on the anteroposterior [AP] film), layering seen with decubitus films if the effusion is free flowing

TABLE 9-1   Evaluation of Pleural Fluid

Test	Transudate	Exudate	Empyema
WBC	<1000	>1000	>10,000 >50,000 most specific
pH	7.45–7.55	≤7.45	<7.30
Pleural fluid protein to serum ratio	<0.5	>0.5	>0.5
Pleural fluid LDH to serum ratio	<0.6	>0.6	>0.6

- CT scan: Detects small effusions (as little as 10 mL). Helps distinguish pleural thickening from effusions, and visualizes underlying lung parenchyma
- **Pleural fluid studies:** Complete blood count (CBC), protein, lactate dehydrogenase (LDH), Gram stain, glucose. Add pH and culture if suspect infection, and cytology if possible malignancy. If sending for cytology, send a large volume of pleural fluid. Pleural fluid amylase helpful if concerned about esophageal rupture or pancreatitis.
- See Table 9-1 for interpretation of studies

■ **Management**

• If effusion is a parapneumonic effusion without infected pleural fluid, treat underlying pneumonia with appropriate antibiotics
• Free-flowing parapneumonic effusions with pH < 7.30, positive Gram stain, or frank empyema should be drained with tube thoracostomy (chest tube). If the effusion is loculated or inadequate drainage from chest tube, then surgical approach through video-assisted thoracoscopy (VATS) or standard thoracotomy should be done

■ **Complications**

• Sepsis and severe pleural scarring

Community-Acquired Pneumonia

Acute pulmonary infection acquired when not hospitalized or in a long-term care facility within the previous 14 days

■ **Epidemiology**

• Sixth most common cause of death in US

- Estimated 2–4 million cases of community-acquired pneumonia (CAP) annually in US, resulting in 500,000 hospitalizations and 45,000 deaths
- Patients over 65 are three to four times more likely to be hospitalized

■ Risk Factors

- Age
- Immunosuppression (HIV, pharmacologic, malignancy)
- Alcohol use
- Impaired swallowing (stroke or other neurologic disease)

■ Etiology

- 40% to 60% of cases have no definite pathogen identified

S. pneumoniae (Pneumococcus)

- Gram-positive diplococcus
- **Accounts for $2/3$ of bacteremic pneumonias**
- More common in elderly and immunocompromised
- Pneumococcal polysaccharide vaccine (PPV; Pneumovax) reduces rates of bacteremia but not pneumonia
- Resistance to beta-lactams and macrolides increasing

"Atypical" Pathogens

- *Mycoplasma pneumoniae*, *Chlamydia pneumoniae*, and *Legionella pneumophila* are significant pathogens
- Difficult to distinguish from typical pathogens by clinical presentation
- No response to beta-lactam antibiotics, good response to macrolides and fluoroquinolones
- ***Legionella* often causes more severe clinical presentation** than *Mycoplasma* or *Chlamydia*, also favors sicker hosts (chronic lung disease, immunosuppressed)

Viruses

- Influenza, hantavirus, and the sudden acute respiratory syndrome (SARS) coronavirus are the most severe but many other viruses can also cause pneumonia
- Difficult to distinguish viral from bacterial pneumonia solely by clinical presentation; exposure history is key

■ Pathogenesis

- Most often caused by inhalation of pathogen from air or colonized oropharynx
- Compromise of host defenses important in pathogenesis
- Can also be seeded hematogenously (e.g., septic emboli in tricuspid valve endocarditis)

■ **History**
- Fever, cough, dyspnea, sputum production, chest pain
- Exposure history (sick contacts, animals)
- Comorbid diseases

■ **Physical Exam**
- Auscultation: **Crackles,** bronchial breath sounds
- Percussion: Dullness over affected lung
- Specific maneuvers
  - **Egophony:** E to A changes over affected lung
  - Tactile fremitus: Palpable vibration over affected lung with provocation; have patient say "toy boat"
  - **Whispered pectoriloquy:** Whispered vocalization heard more clearly over affected lung

■ **Additional Studies**
- Oximetry (or blood gas if severely ill)
- Complete blood count, chemistry panel
- CXR: Usually shows opacity in affected lung, may be lobar consolidation or diffuse interstitial infiltrates
- Sputum Gram stain and culture
  - Use is controversial
  - Gram stain may be useful if high quality: Fewer than 10 epithelial cells and more than 25 WBCs per low-power field, and a dominant pathogen
  - Culture valuable if suspected drug resistance (e.g., pneumococci, gram-negative rods)
- Blood cultures: If positive, may help with pathogen identification
- HIV testing if risk factors present
- **Specific *Legionella* testing (sputum culture or urinary antigen) if severely ill**
- Isolation and tuberculosis testing if risk factors present

■ **Differential Diagnosis**
- Acute bronchitis: Should not have abnormal CXR or hypoxemia (except in chronic lung disease)
- Pulmonary embolism: Can present with dyspnea, fever, hemoptysis, chest pain, hypoxia; CXR usually normal or only mildly abnormal
- CHF: Can present with dyspnea, hemoptysis, hypoxia, chest pain, bilateral infiltrates on CXR; should not have fever or leukocytosis. Look for other signs/symptoms of CHF (orthopnea, edema, elevated neck veins)
- Lung cancer: Can cause recurrent pneumonia because of airway obstruction, or an infiltrate that appears to be pneumonia but doesn't resolve

■ TABLE 9-2	Empiric Treatment of CAP	
Treatment Group	Option 1	Option 2
Low-risk outpatient	Azithromycin	Doxycycline
Higher-risk outpatient	Beta-lactam[a] + azithromycin	Fluoroquinolone[b]
Low-risk inpatient	IV azithromycin ± IV beta-lactam[c]	IV or oral fluoroquinolone[b]
High-risk inpatient	IV beta-lactam[c] + either IV azithromycin or IV fluoroquinolone	

[a] For example, amoxicillin, amoxicillin/clavulanate, cefpodoxime
[b] For example, levofloxacin, sparfloxacin, moxifloxacin, gatifloxacin, see comment Table 3.3
[c] For example, ampicillin/sulbactam, ceftriaxone, cefotaxime

■ Management

Initial Triage

- Consider hospital admission in patients with one or more risk factors:
  - Hypoxemia
  - Hypotension, tachycardia, tachypnea
  - Age over 65 years
  - Comorbid illness (cardiopulmonary disease, renal failure, diabetes, chronic liver disease, alcohol abuse, cerebrovascular disease, malnutrition, splenectomy)
  - Multilobar or cavitary pneumonia
  - Pleural effusion
  - WBC < 4,000 or > 30,000; hematocrit < 30%; creatinine > 1.2; pH < 7.35
  - Poor social situation

Outpatient Management

- Patients with good support at home, the ability to follow up quickly, and few or no risk factors may be better managed as outpatients
- Prediction rules exist to facilitate decision making
- See Table 9-2 for treatment options
  - Low-risk outpatient: No cardiopulmonary disease or risk factors for specific organisms
  - Higher-risk outpatient: Comorbid cardiopulmonary disease or other risk factors

Inpatient Management

- See Table 9-2 for treatment options
  - Low-risk inpatient: Meets criteria for admission but few risk factors

  - High-risk inpatient: Multiple risk factors, intensive care unit admission
- Patients with structural lung disease (bronchiectasis, cystic fibrosis) should be treated with antipseudomonal antibiotics (see below, "Nosocomial Pneumonia")

■ Complications
- Pleural effusion, empyema, lung abscess, sepsis

Nosocomial Pneumonia

Defined as **pneumonia occurring 48 hours or more after hospital admission,** but broadly includes patients in long-term care facilities

■ Epidemiology
- Estimated 5–10 cases per 1000 admissions

■ Risk Factors
- Mechanical ventilation (6- to 20-fold increased risk)
- Prolonged hospitalization
- Antibiotic use
- Corticosteroid use
- Nasogastric tube
- H_2 blocker or antacid use
- Altered mental status
- Age over 70 years
- Comorbid diseases: COPD, diabetes, alcoholism, renal insufficiency, cigarette smoking, respiratory failure

■ Etiology
- Gram-negative rods: *Pseudomonas aeruginosa, Enterobacter* spp, *Klebsiella* spp, *Escherichia coli, Serratia marcescens, Haemophilus influenzae, Acinetobacter* spp
- *S. aureus*
- Anaerobes
- *Legionella* spp
- Fungi
- Many pathogens have resistance to multiple antibiotics

■ Pathogenesis
- Compromised host defenses
  - Endotracheal tube provides direct conduit to lower respiratory tract, also site of microbial colonization
  - Corticosteroids
  - Acute illness

- Altered microbial flora: Multiple resistant organisms are endemic in medical care facilities because of antibiotic use. Patient exposure to antibiotics selects for these organisms
- Aspiration: Aspiration of gastric contents plays a greater role in nosocomial pneumonia than CAP. Increasing gastric pH for ulcer prophylaxis may increase risk of pneumonia

■ History
- Fever, cough, dyspnea, chest pain, purulent sputum production
- Decreased oxygenation/increased requirement for supplemental oxygen
- Consider risk factors listed above

■ Physical Exam
- See Community-Acquired Pneumonia, above

■ Additional Studies
- Oximetry/blood gas
- Complete blood cell count, chemistry panel
- CXR: Opacity in affected lung, may be lobar consolidation or diffuse interstitial infiltrates. May be more difficult to interpret in hospitalized patients because of non-infectious CXR abnormalities (e.g., atelectasis, acute respiratory distress syndrome [ARDS])
- Sputum Gram stain and culture
- Gram stain useful if there is a dominant pathogen
- Culture helpful in tailoring antibiotic therapy, as **resistance is often an issue**
- Fungal cultures if suspicion (immunosuppression, prolonged antibiotic or corticosteroid use)
- Blood cultures may help with identification of pathogen
- *Legionella* testing (culture or urinary antigen) if severely ill
- Consider more invasive pulmonary culture (bronchoalveolar lavage or protected brush sampling) if above doesn't yield an organism and nosocomial pneumonia still suspected

■ Differential Diagnosis
- Other causes of fever in hospitalized patient: Urinary tract infection (UTI), sinusitis, wound infection, deep venous thrombosis (DVT), *Clostridium difficile* colitis, occult abscess, drug reaction
- Other causes of decreased oxygenation: Pulmonary embolism, CHF, ARDS
- Other causes of abnormal CXR: Atelectasis, CHF, ARDS

■ **TABLE 9-3   Specific Risk Factors and Suggested Management in Nosocomial Pneumonia**

Risk Factor	Organism	Antibiotic
Recent abdominal surgery, witnessed aspiration	Anaerobes	Clindamycin or beta-lactam/ beta-lactamase inhibitor
Coma, head trauma, diabetes, renal failure	*S. aureus*	Vancomycin (until MRSA no longer a concern)
High-dose steroids	*Legionella* spp	Erythromycin
Structural lung disease, steroids, antibiotic use	*P. aeruginosa*	Treat as for severe pneumonia

Abbreviations: MRSA, methicillin-resistant *S. aureus*

■ **Management**

General Principles
- Antibiotic therapy should be directed against prevalent organisms at the hospital/long-term care facility
- Consider antibiotic exposure and expand coverage if needed
- Cautious interpretation of culture results when available can help to narrow antibiotic coverage
- **Specific risk factors require broader coverage** (Table 9-3)

Mild to Moderate Pneumonia, No Risk Factors
- Penicillin/beta-lactamase inhibitor (e.g., ampicillin/sulbactam), or
- Second- or third-generation cephalosporin (e.g., ceftriaxone), or
- Fluoroquinolone (e.g., levofloxacin)
- Consider using antipseudomonal agent if patient was previously on antibiotics

Severe Pneumonia
- Antipseudomonal beta-lactam
  - Antipseudomonal penicillin (e.g., piperacillin) ± beta-lactamase inhibitor, or
  - Antipseudomonal cephalosporin (e.g., ceftazidime), or
  - Carbapenem (e.g., imipenem)
- Combine the above beta-lactam with expanded gram-negative agent
  - Aminoglycoside (e.g., tobramycin)
  - Fluoroquinolone (e.g., ciprofloxacin)
- Add vancomycin if suspected MRSA

■ **Complications**
- Pleural effusion, empyema, lung abscess, sepsis, extended hospital stay

Tuberculosis

■ Epidemiology

- US incidence declined between 1953 and 1985, increased between 1985 and 1992
- Excess cases likely due to HIV
- Increased rates of primary tuberculosis (TB)
- Increased rates of multidrug-resistant (MDR) TB
- Incidence in sub-Saharan Africa, India, China, southeast Asia is high and expected to rise because of HIV

■ Risk Factors

- HIV infection
- Homelessness
- Incarceration
- Injection drug use
- Health care workers
- Emigrants from high-prevalence countries

■ Etiology and Pathogenesis

- *Mycobacterium tuberculosis* grows slowly in culture and can be seen microscopically only with acid-fast staining. Also known as acid-fast bacilli (AFB)
- Usual portal of entry is through inhalation
- Initial infection may manifest as primary pulmonary TB with presentation similar to pneumonia
- Host immune response usually suppresses clinical manifestations in immunocompetent hosts (latent TB)
- Patients with latent TB infection have a positive tuberculin skin test but not active TB
- Latent TB **reactivates in approximately 10% of patients**
- Reactivation TB frequently presents in the lungs but may also involve other sites: Pleural space, bone, gastrointestinal tract, meninges, eye, genitourinary tract, peritoneum, lymph nodes
- **Miliary TB** refers to widely disseminated TB with multiple sites of involvement; clinical manifestations are variable and nonspecific

■ History

- Cough, chest pain, **hemoptysis**
- **Weight loss,** fever, fatigue, **night sweats**
- History of known TB exposure
- History of positive tuberculin skin test (PPD)
- Positive risk factors

■ **Physical Exam**

• Fever, **cachexia,** lymphadenopathy
• Crackles, **apical hyperresonance** (if cavitary disease)
• Dullness to percussion if pleural effusion present

■ **Additional Studies**

• CXR
  - **Apical infiltrates** present in 70% to 90% of reactivation TB
  - **Cavitary lesions** present in 20% to 40% of reactivation TB
  - Primary TB may appear similar to pneumonia
  - **Hilar adenopathy** common, especially among HIV patients
  - **Calcified granulomata** suggest previous TB exposure, nondiagnostic for active disease
• Sputum AFB stain and culture
  - Useful to confirm diagnosis and assess need for isolation
  - Three negative AFB smears on expectorated sputa are sufficient to remove patient from isolation
  - One to three induced sputa can be used instead of expectorated sputa if patient isn't coughing
  - Culture is more sensitive than smear. Culture is also valuable in assessing antibiotic resistance
• Tuberculin PPD skin test
  - Essential in diagnosis of latent TB, unreliable in active TB
  - Intradermal injection, read by diameter of induration at injection site between 48 and 72 hours
  - Diameter of induration considered positive varies from 5 mm to 15 mm based on risk factors (Table 9-4)

■ **Differential Diagnosis**

• Sarcoidosis, histoplasmosis, malignancy, nontuberculous mycobacterial infection

■ **TABLE 9-4** Threshold for Positive PPD Skin Tests Based on Risk Factors		
Induration ≥ 5 mm	**Induration ≥ 10 mm**	**Induration ≥ 15 mm**
HIV-positive	Recent (<5 yr) emigrant from high-prevalence country	No other risk factors for TB
Known TB exposure	Injection drug use	
CXR suggestive of prior TB exposure	Homeless, incarcerated, other high-risk settings	
Immunosuppression	Healthcare workers	
	Children exposed to high-risk adults	

■ Management

Latent TB

- Isoniazid (INH) daily for 9 months is preferred regimen
- INH daily for 6 months acceptable in HIV-negative patients
- Either INH regimen can be given as twice-weekly directly observed therapy (DOT) instead of daily
- Rifampin daily for 4 months is backup in patients with known INH-resistant exposure
- Rifampin-pyrazinamide (RIF-PZA) 2-month course was popular briefly but no longer recommended because of hepatotoxicity

Active TB

- Active TB requires 6–9 months of multidrug therapy
- Regular completion of all doses is essential; DOT is preferred, especially in high-risk patients
- Multiple possible regimens: all start with a 2-month phase of four drugs: INH, rifampin (RIF), ethambutol (EMB), and pyrazinamide (PZA)
- EMB is stopped if testing confirms INH-sensitive organism
- Sputum AFB smear and culture repeated at 2 months
- Regimens then continue for 4 months, usually with INH-RIF combination either daily or twice weekly
- Patients with cavitary disease and positive 2-month culture receive 7 months of INH-RIF (total 9 months of therapy)
- HIV-negative patients with negative smear at 2 months can use once-weekly regimen of INH-rifapentine

■ Complications

- Lung cavitation, pneumothorax, disseminated TB

Cardiac Infections

Melissa M. Hagman, MD

Endocarditis

Inflammation of endocardium (most commonly heart valves)

■ Epidemiology
- Native heart valves
  - 1.7–6.2 cases per 100,000 person-years in the US
  - 70% of patients have underlying structural heart abnormality
- Prosthetic heart valves
  - Approximately one case per 100,000 person-years
  - Mechanical valves are at higher risk in **first 1–2 months;** at 5 years, risks similar for mechanical and bioprostheses
- Injection drug users (IDU): 150–200 (cases per 100,000) person-years
- Nosocomial: Incidence unknown, fatality rate ~50%

■ Risk Factors
(See Chapter 21 for endocarditis prophylaxis)
- **Valvular heart disease,** prosthetic valve, IDU, poor dental hygiene, hemodialysis, **indwelling central venous catheter,** recent procedures (dental, urologic, gynecologic, gastrointestinal, etc.)

■ Etiology
- Native valves (Table 10-1)
- Prosthetic valves
  - Early infection (2 months or less after surgery): *S. aureus,* **coagulase-negative staphylococci**
  - Late infection (over 12 months): Same as native valve disease
- IDU: Skin flora, often methicillin-resistant *S. aureus* (MRSA)
- Nosocomial: *S. aureus,* coagulase-negative staphylococci

■ Pathogenesis
- Blood-borne pathogens adhere to the endocardium (especially abnormal heart valves) and cause local tissue injury, vegetation formation, and embolization

■ TABLE 10-1	Pathogens in Native Valve Endocarditis
Culture Positive	**Culture Negative[a]**
Staphylococcus aureus	HACEK[b]
Streptococcus spp (S. bovis often associated with gastrointestinal malignancy)	Bartonella spp (B. quintana associated with homelessness, chronic alcohol use; transmitted by body lice; diagnosed by serology)
Enterococcus spp	Abiotrophia spp
	Coxiella burnetii (Q fever)
	Chlamydia spp
	Tropheryma whipplei
	Legionella spp
	Brucella spp
	Fungi

[a] 5% to 7% of cases if no antibiotics given before cultures are drawn
[b] Haemophilus spp, Actinobacillus actinomycetemcomitans, Cardiobacterium hominis, Eikenella corrodens, Kingella kingae

■ **History**

- Less-virulent organisms (e.g., viridans streptococci): **Insidious onset of fatigue,** malaise, anorexia, weight loss, arthralgias
- More-virulent organisms (e.g., *S. aureus*): Often present dramatically with **fever and rigors**

■ **Physical Exam**

- Cardiac signs
  - Preexisting murmur suggesting predisposing disease
  - Regurgitant murmur suggesting new valvular insufficiency
- Embolic signs
  - **Conjunctival hemorrhages**
  - **Janeway lesions:** Nontender, erythematous, hemorrhagic lesions on palms or soles
- Immunologic signs
  - **Osler's nodes:** Tender subcutaneous nodules on hands or feet
  - **Roth's spots:** Round, white retinal spots surrounded by hemorrhage

■ **Diagnosis**

Modified Duke criteria (Box 10-1)

■ **BOX 10-1 Modified Duke Criteria for Diagnosis of Infective Endocarditis**

Major Criteria

Typical organism (e.g., *S. aureus*, streptococci) from two BCs

Any organism grown from persistently positive BC

Positive serologic test or single BC for *C. burnetii* (Q fever)

Echocardiogram showing oscillating intracardiac mass, abscess, or new dehiscence of prosthetic valve

Physical exam showing new valvular regurgitation (change in preexisting murmur not sufficient)

Minor Criteria

Predisposing heart condition or injection drug use

Fever (temperature over 100.4°F [38.0°C])

Vascular phenomena (e.g., major arterial emboli, septic pulmonary infarcts, mycotic aneurysm, intracranial hemorrhage, conjunctival hemorrhages, Janeway lesions [petechiae or splinter hemorrhages not sufficient])

Immunologic phenomena (e.g., glomerulonephritis, Osler's nodes, Roth's spots, positive rheumatoid factor)

Serologic evidence or positive BC not meeting a major criterion

Diagnosis

Definite endocarditis: Either two major, one major + three minor, or five minor criteria

Possible endocarditis: Either one major + one minor, or three minor criteria

Abbreviations: BC, blood culture

■ **Additional Studies**

- Lab tests
  - Blood cultures before antibiotics are vital for diagnosis and antibiotic susceptibility testing, alert lab if HACEK or other fastidious organisms suspected
  - Serology in selected cases (e.g., *Bartonella*)
  - Complete blood count: Often shows **anemia** and leukocytosis
  - Urinalysis: **Hematuria** may indicate glomerulonephritis
- Electrocardiogram (ECG): May show PR prolongation from complication of perivalvular abscess
- Chest x-ray (CXR): Evidence of **septic lung emboli** sometimes present in right-sided endocarditis
- Echocardiogram: Usually necessary for diagnosis
  - Transthoracic echocardiogram (TTE): Good initial study

- Transesophageal echocardiogram (TEE): Pursue if TTE negative. **TEE more sensitive** for vegetations, abscesses, and perivalvular leaks

Differential Diagnosis
- Acute rheumatic fever, atrial myxoma, collagen vascular disease (e.g., systemic lupus erythematosus [SLE])

Management
- Antimicrobials
  - Empiric therapy: **Vancomycin ± gentamicin**
  - Subsequent therapy driven by culture results (Table 10-2)
- Indications for **surgical management**
  - Congestive heart failure (CHF)
  - Perivalvular extension of infection
  - Microbiologic failure (i.e., inability to clear blood cultures)
  - Infection with fungi or untreatable pathogens
  - One or two major emboli with residual large mobile vegetation

Complications
- Conduction abnormalities, CHF, vertebral osteomyelitis, emboli to brain/spleen/kidneys, septic arthritis, **mycotic aneurysms**

Myocarditis

Nonischemic inflammation of heart muscle

Epidemiology
- Cause of approximately 20% of sudden cardiac deaths in autopsied adults under 40 years of age
- May account for 10% of unexplained cases of heart failure

Risk Factors
- Immunocompromised states (e.g., HIV)

Etiology
- Often unknown
- Most common: Viruses (e.g., **coxsackievirus B,** adenovirus, influenza virus, hepatitis C virus, cytomegalovirus, parvovirus)
- Less common: Bacteria (usually in setting of abscess extension from endocarditis), spirochetes, fungi, protozoa (e.g., *Trypanosoma cruzi* in Chagas' disease), parasites, rickettsiae

■ TABLE 10-2   Management of Endocarditis

Culture-Positive

Native Valve	Prosthetic Valve
Streptococci (penicillin MIC < 0.1 µg/mL)	
4 weeks penicillin OR 2 weeks penicillin + LD gentamicin	6 weeks penicillin + LD gentamicin for the first 2 weeks
Streptococci (penicillin MIC 0.1–0.5 µg/mL)	
4 weeks penicillin + gentamicin for the first 2 weeks	6 weeks penicillin + LD gentamicin for the first 2–4 weeks
Streptococci (penicillin MIC > 0.5 µg/mL) or Enterococci	
4 weeks penicillin + LD gentamicin	Penicillin + LD gentamicin for 6 weeks
Methicillin-susceptible staphylococci	
4–6 weeks nafcillin + LD gentamicin for first 3–5 days	6 weeks nafcillin + oral rifampin (added after a few days) + LD gentamicin for the first 2 weeks
Methicillin-resistant staphylococci	
4–6 weeks vancomycin + LD gentamicin for the first 3–5 days	6 weeks vancomycin + oral rifampin (added after a few days) + LD gentamicin for first 2 week s
HACEK microorganisms	
4 weeks ceftriaxone OR 4 weeks ampicillin + LD gentamicin	6 weeks ceftriaxone OR 6 weeks ampicillin + LD gentamicin

Culture-Negative

Native Valve	Prosthetic Valve
Varies; consider 4 weeks vancomycin + LD gentamicin (can add ceftriaxone for HACEK coverage)	Varies; consider 6 weeks vancomycin + LD gentamicin (can add ceftriaxone for HACEK coverage)

Abbreviations: LD, low-dose (1 mg/kg every 8 hours; target peak > 3 µg/mL); MIC, minimal inhibitory concentration; HACEK, *Haemophilus* spp., *Actinobacillus actinomycetemcomitans, Cardiobacterium hominis, Eikenella corrodens,* and *Kingella kingae* hepatitis A virus

■ Pathogenesis

- Viruses: Patchy lymphocytic infiltrates and myocyte necrosis
- Bacterial and parasitic pathogens: Neutrophilic infiltrates, abscesses, and granulomas
- Chagas' disease: Trypanosomes parasitize myocytes and produce eosinophilic inflammation

■ History

- Often asymptomatic
- **Nonpleuritic chest pain,** fatigue, dyspnea

- Viral prodrome of fever and myalgias with or without recent upper respiratory tract illness or enteritis

■ **Physical Exam**
- Often normal
- Fever and hemodynamic instability in fulminant cases
- Signs of **CHF** (S_3, crackles on lung exam, elevated neck veins)
- Pericardial rub may be present if pericardium also involved

■ **Additional Studies**
- Lab tests
  - WBC: Often elevated, possible lymphocytosis or eosinophilia
  - Cardiac enzymes: Elevated with myonecrosis
- ECG: Usually normal. May show sinus tachycardia, ventricular arrhythmias, heart block, or changes mimicking acute myocardial infarction (MI) or pericarditis
- Endomyocardial biopsy: May show white blood cell **infiltrates**. Sensitivity of biopsy as low as 35%
- Identification of offending viruses (often unsuccessful)
  - PCR of biopsy specimens for presence of viral genome
  - Viral cultures (from stool, pharyngeal washings, other fluids)
  - Acute and convalescent antibody titers
- Echocardiography: Assesses ventricular function

■ **Differential Diagnosis**
- Noninfectious myocarditis
- Immune-mediated (e.g., sarcoidosis, scleroderma, SLE, other rheumatologic conditions)
- Toxic (e.g., ethanol, cocaine, anthracyclines, heavy metals, electric shock, radiation, hyperpyrexia, snake or spider bites, bee stings)

■ **Management**
- Supportive care for CHF (diuretics, angiotensin-converting enzyme inhibitors, beta-blockers, vasodilators, etc.)
  - Fulminant cases may require intravenous inotropes, intraaortic balloon pump, or left ventricular assist devices
- Telemetry monitoring
  - **Treat arrhythmias/heart block:** Drugs, defibrillation, or pacing
- Limited physical activity for acute stages of disease
- Antiviral therapy (e.g., ribavirin or interferon) may be of benefit, but clinical data are sparse
- Immunosuppression not proved beneficial

■ **Complications**
- Most cases resolve spontaneously without further sequelae. However, some progress to dilated cardiomyopathy years later
- Fulminant cases with rapid onset of heart failure often result either in swift progression to death or full spontaneous recovery
- Ventricular or atrial arrhythmias can occur in the acute phase

Pericarditis

Inflammation of the pericardium

■ **Epidemiology**
- Accounts for ~5% of non-MI chest pain in emergency room patients

■ **Risk Factors**
- Immunocompromised states, trauma, infection of contiguous organs or spaces

■ **Etiology**
- Undetermined in ~30% of cases
- Viral causes are most common (Table 10-3)

■ **Pathogenesis**
- Pathogens spread to pericardium hematogenously or from contiguous organs and cause inflammation
- Viruses produce serous pericarditis with small amounts of pericardial fluid and lymphocytic pericardial inflammation

■ TABLE 10-3	Causes of Infectious Pericarditis
Pathogens	**Organisms**
Viruses	Coxsackievirus, echovirus, adenovirus, influenza, mumps, varicella
	Herpes simplex and cytomegalovirus in immunocompromised hosts
Bacteria	*Staphylococcus* and *Streptococcus* most often
	Other pathogens include those from concurrent bacteremia, pneumonia, or mediastinal infection (especially if the infection has extended beyond the pericardial barrier)
Mycobacteria	*M. tuberculosis* in developing countries
	M. avium-intracellulare complex in immunocompromised hosts
Fungi	*Histoplasma capsulatum, Cryptococcus neoformans*
Parasites	Toxoplasmosis, Chagas' disease

- Bacteria, fungi, and parasites cause purulent pericarditis with granular changes to the epi- and pericardial surfaces
- **M. tuberculosis** (as well as malignancy, uremia, or trauma) causes **hemorrhagic pericarditis**

■ History

- Acute presentation: **Sharp pleuritic, anterior chest pain** that radiates to back, trapezius ridge, neck and jaw; pain worsens when supine; fever may be present
- Subacute/chronic presentation: Chest pain uncommon, only symptoms may be from complications (e.g., **shortness of breath from tamponade** or constrictive pericarditis)
- Systemic symptoms of underlying disease may be present (e.g., weight loss with *M. tuberculosis*; rhinorrhea, malaise, and myalgias with viral syndrome)

■ Physical Exam

- **Pericardial rub:** Heard best at left sternal border in end expiration with patient leaning forward

■ Additional Studies

- ECG: **Most helpful test,** changes evolve over days to weeks
  - Stage I (early): Diffuse, upwardly concave ST-segment elevation and PR-segment depression
  - Stage II: Near normalization of ECG
  - Stage III (resolving): Diffuse T wave inversions
  - Stage IV: Normalization of ECG
  - Low voltage or electrical alternans with pericardial effusions
  - Atrial arrhythmias (e.g., flutter or fibrillation) occur rarely
- CXR: **Enlarged cardiac silhouette** if pericardial effusion present
- Lab tests
  - WBC: Often elevated, granulocytosis, then lymphocytosis
  - Cardiac enzymes: May be elevated
  - Other tests to consider include blood cultures, metabolic panel to assess for uremia, rheumatoid factor, antinuclear antibody, viral studies, and tuberculin skin testing
- Echocardiography, computed tomogram (CT), and magnetic resonance imaging (MRI): Helpful in assessing for effusion or constriction; not necessary in uncomplicated cases
- **Pericardiocentesis:** Indicated in clinical tamponade, purulent pericarditis, and when tumor is suspected (Box 10-2)
- Pericardial biopsy: Helpful in *M. tuberculosis* or malignancy

■ Differential Diagnosis

- MI, aortic dissection, pulmonary embolism, pneumonia, empyema, pneumothorax

▓ BOX 10-2   Pericardial Fluid Testing for Pericarditis of Unknown Etiology

Always
Glucose

Protein

Lactate dehydrogenase

Cell count and differential

Gram stain

Bacterial culture

Cytology

Sometimes
Viral culture

Adenosine dehydrogenase (present in *M. tuberculosis*)

PCR for viruses or *M. tuberculosis*

Immunohistochemistry for antibodies to myolemma and sarcolemma (immune-mediated pericarditis)

Carcinoembryonic antigen (>5 ng/mL; 75% sensitivity and 100% specificity for neoplasm)

- Noninfectious causes of pericarditis: Trauma, metabolic derangements (especially uremia and myxedema), malignancy, rheumatologic disorders, post-MI, drugs

▓ Management
- Idiopathic and viral pericarditis
    - Supportive, course usually benign (lasting 3–6 weeks)
    - **Nonsteroidal anti-inflammatory drugs (NSAIDs):** First-line therapy
    - Colchicine: Used for NSAID nonresponders
- Bacterial, fungal, parasitic pericarditis
    - Antimicrobials
    - Consider drainage of any effusion
- Steroid use is controversial
    - Decreases risk of constriction with *M. tuberculosis*
    - May increase risk of chronic relapsing pericarditis

▓ Complications
- **Recurrent pericarditis** (up to **30% of patients**), pericardial constriction, cardiac tamponade

Gastrointestinal Infections

Peggy D. Headstrom, MD

Hepatitis A Virus

■ Epidemiology

- The most common cause of viral hepatitis
- In the US, the seroprevalence rate is 38%; rates increase with age
- Living conditions of poor sanitation and hygiene
- Group living situations
- Daycare centers, military camps, institutions

■ Pathogenesis

- RNA virus from the family Picornaviridae
- Person-to-person transmission via the **fecal-oral** route

■ History/Physical Exam

- Incubation period is 15–50 days
- Symptomatic or asymptomatic
- Prodromal symptoms include: Fatigue, weakness, anorexia, nausea, vomiting, abdominal pain
- Jaundice, dark urine, and acholic stools occur within 1–2 weeks of prodromal symptoms
- **Right upper quadrant tenderness** and mild liver enlargement are seen in 85% of patients
- Less common findings include splenomegaly, cervical lymphadenopathy, and rash

■ Additional Studies

- Serum **aminotransferases** (ALT and AST) increase during prodromal phase
- Bilirubin peaks after the peak in aminotransferases and falls more slowly
- IgM anti-HAV detection in serum is gold standard for diagnosis
- IgG anti-HAV indicate previous exposure and immunity to HAV

■ Management

- Generally a self-limited acute infection
- Symptomatic treatment

■ **Prevention**
- Pooled human immune globulin provides passive protection
- Given to **household contacts** within 1–2 weeks of exposure or prior to **travel** in endemic areas
- Vaccine of inactivated virus with close to 100% seroconversion rate after two doses

■ **Complications**
- Fulminant hepatitis is rare
- Associated with underlying liver disease and older age

Hepatitis B Virus

■ **Epidemiology**
- Global prevalence of 300 million carriers (5% of world population)
- High prevalence areas include Asia, Africa, Middle East, and parts of South America
- HBV can cause **acute or chronic** infection
  - Chronic infection occurs after an acute infection in 5% of adult population
  - Very high risk of chronic infection in neonates

■ **Risk Factors**
- In the US, injection drug users and men who have sex with men (MSM) are at highest risk
- Sexual partners of HBV-infected carriers
- Healthcare workers
- Patients on hemodialysis
- Children born to mothers who are infected

■ **Etiology**
- Partly double-stranded DNA virus in the family Hepadnaviridae

■ **Transmission**
- Parenteral transmission
- Sexual transmission
- Perinatal or vertical transmission

■ **History/Physical Exam**
- History and physical exam of acute infection may resemble hepatitis A infection
- Acute or chronic infection may be asymptomatic
- Acute infection has an incubation period of 60–180 days

■ TABLE 11-1   Hepatitis B Serologic Markers and Disease States

	HBsAg	HBsAb	HBcAb IgM	HBcAb IgG	HBeAg	HBeAb	HBVDNA
Acute	+	−	+	−	+	−	+
Chronic active	+	−	−	+/−	+	−	+
Healthy carrier	+	−	−	+	−	+	−
Resolved	−	+	−	+	−	+	−
Vaccinated	−	+	−	−	−	−	−

Abbreviations: HBcAb, antibody to hepatitis B core antigen; HBeAb, antibody to hepatitis B envelope antigen; HBeAg, hepatitis B envelope antigen; HBsAb, antibody to hepatitis B surface antigen; HBsAg, hepatitis B surface antigen; HBV DNA, hepatitis B virus deoxyribonucleic acid

■ Additional Studies

• HBV serological markers can be used to distinguish between HBV disease states (Table 11-1)

■ Management

• No treatment for acute HBV in immunocompetent adults
• Moderate to severe chronic hepatitis
  - Interferon, lamivudine, adefovir have all been approved

■ Prevention

• Behavior modification
• Active immunization
  - Antibodies to HBV develop in 95% of recipients

■ Complications

• Cirrhosis
• Hepatocellular carcinoma
• Polyarteritis nodosa
• Membranous glomerulonephropathy

Hepatitis C Virus

■ Epidemiology

• 3–4 million people in the US infected
• 2.7 million people with chronic infection
• The most common chronic blood-borne infection in the US

■ Risk Factors

• Injection drug use is the most common risk factor

- Blood transfusion prior to 1992, unsafe medical practices, birth to an infected mother, sexual transmission (increased risk with multiple sexual partners)

■ Etiology

- RNA virus in the family Flaviviridae
- Six different genotypes
- Genotype 1 accounts for 70% to 75% of HCV infections in US

■ Transmission

- Exposure to blood products
- Vertical transmission
- Sexual transmission

■ History/Physical Exam

- Acute infection
  - Incubation period 6–7 weeks
  - Symptoms develop in only 25% to 35% of patients
  - Nonspecific vague symptoms in 10% to 20% of patients
  - Jaundice in 25% of patients
- Chronic infection develops in **85%** of infected patients
  - **Fatigue** is the most common symptom
  - Jaundice is rarely seen

■ Additional Studies

- Acute infection
  - ALT may rise during this period
  - HCV RNA present within 2 weeks of exposure
- Chronic infection
  - Fluctuating ALT, one-third of patients will have normal ALT
- Anti-HCV test
  - Enzyme immunosorbent assay (EIA) to detect hepatitis C antibodies
  - 99% sensitivity in immunocompetent patients
- Quantitative HCV RNA assay
  - Gives information of viral load
  - Little correlation between disease activity and viral level
  - Provides information on response to treatment
- Liver biopsy: Provides information on degree of fibrosis

■ Prevention

- No vaccine available
- Behavior modification

■ Management

- Interferon and ribavirin

- Genotype 1 patients achieved a sustained virological response rate of 43% to 46%
- Genotype 2 and 3 patients achieved a sustained virological response rate of 76% to 82%

■ Complications

- Cirrhosis in 10% to 15% of chronically infected patients
- Hepatocellular carcinoma
- **Extrahepatic manifestations:** Essential mixed cryoglobulinemia, glomerulonephritis, keratoconjunctivitis sicca, lichen planus, lymphoma, porphyria cutanea tarda

Hepatitis D Virus (HDV)

- Presence of **HBV is necessary** for infection
- Increased risk of **cirrhosis or fulminant hepatitis** if **coinfected** with hepatitis D and HBV compared with HBV alone

Hepatitis E Virus

- Cause of **acute hepatitis,** especially in developing countries
- Fecal-oral transmission
- Similar clinical course to hepatitis A
- Particularly severe in third trimester of **pregnancy**

Infectious Diarrhea

■ Epidemiology

- Acute diarrhea is three or more watery stools a day for less than 14 days
- The second most common cause of death worldwide
- In the US, 211 million to 375 million episodes of acute diarrhea each year
- Risk factors are young age, ingestion of contaminated food, daycare or institution worker or resident

■ Etiology

- **Bacterial:** Toxigenic (enterotoxin-producing) versus invasive
- **Toxigenic:** *Vibrio cholerae*, enterotoxigenic *Escherichia coli* (ETEC), enteropathogenic *E. coli* (EPEC), enterohemorrhagic *E. coli* (EHEC), *Aeromonas*
- **Invasive:**
  - Organism penetrates the mucosal surface
  - *Salmonella, Shigella*, enteroinvasive *E. coli* (EIEC), *Campylobacter,* and *Yersinia*

- **Viral:** Rotavirus, enteric adenovirus, calicivirus, astrovirus, Norwalk virus, coronavirus
- **Protozoa and parasites:** *Entamoeba histolytica*, *Giardia lamblia*, *Isospora*, *Cyclospora*, *Microsporidium*, and *Cryptosporidium*

■ Pathogenesis

- Increased intestinal secretion of fluid and electrolytes via secretory enterotoxins
- Decreased intestinal absorption due to intestinal epithelial injury

■ History

- Onset of illness, duration of symptoms, weight loss, nocturnal symptoms, sick contacts, fever, nausea, abdominal pain, fecal urgency, tenesmus
- **Vomiting:** Virus, toxin-induced food poisoning (*Staphylococcus aureus*, *Bacillus cereus*, *Clostridium perfringens*)
- Presence of **bloody stool:** *Salmonella*, *Shigella*, *Campylobacter*, and shiga toxin-producing *E. coli* (EHEC)
- **Travel** history: *E. histolytica*
- Exposure to untreated **water:** *Giardia* and *Cryptosporidium*
- Ingestion of **shellfish:** *Vibrio* spp
- Unpasteurized **dairy products** or **undercooked meat:** EHEC
- Timing of symptoms:
  - Symptoms within 6 hours of ingestion of food suggests **preformed toxin:** *S. aureus*, *Bacillus cereus*
  - Symptoms within 8–14 hours suggest *Clostridium perfringens*
  - Symptoms after 14 hours suggest viral etiology, EHEC, or ETEC

■ Physical Exam

- Focus on evidence of **volume depletion** and **systemic toxicity**
  - Fever, tachycardia, hypotension, jugular venous distension
- Abdominal exam: Peritoneal signs suggest an invasive enteric pathogen and may require prompt surgical evaluation

■ Additional Studies

- The frequency of isolating an organism from a stool culture in infectious diarrhea ranges from 2% to 40%
- Most cases of infectious diarrhea are self-limited
- Workup should be pursued in patients with fever, bloody diarrhea, prolonged course, systemic illness, immunocompromised, elderly
- **Fecal leukocytes** (suggest colonic source of infection): *Campylobacter*, *Shigella*, *Salmonella*, EIEC, *Yersinia*
  - Sensitivity 73%, specificity 84%

- Fecal lactoferrin latex agglutination may be more sensitive and specific
- **Stool cultures** if any of the following are present: Severe diarrhea, bloody stools, fever, more than 6 unformed stools/day, diarrhea for longer than 48 hours, severe abdominal pain in patients over 50 years old
  - Useful for patients hospitalized 3 days or less
- **Ova and parasite** (O&P) and *Giardia*-specific antigen: Prolonged diarrhea, immunocompromised, MSM, travel to mountainous regions
- **Endoscopy** (colonoscopy or flexible sigmoidoscopy): Persistent diarrhea, toxic patients

■ Differential Diagnosis

- Inflammatory bowel disease, medication side effect, radiation enteritis, intestinal ischemia, heavy metal ingestion

■ Management

- Rehydration
  - Oral rehydration solution: Mild-moderate diarrhea
  - Intravenous fluids for severely dehydrated patients
- Empiric antibiotics for severe community acquired diarrhea, more than 3 days, with at least one of the following: Abdominal pain, fever, vomiting, myalgia, or headache
  - Treatment with fluoroquinolone for 5 days
  - Shown to reduce duration of symptoms
- Antidiarrheal agents: Loperamide, opiates, bismuth subsalicylate
  - Should be avoided in patients with bloody diarrhea, although limited data supporting this
- Tailor therapy based on cultured organism (Table 11-2)

■ Complications

- EHEC: Hemolytic-uremic syndrome (HUS)
  - Fever, thrombocytopenia, decreased renal function
  - Risk may increase with antibiotic usage
- *Shigella:* Joint inflammation
- *Salmonella:* Meningitis, arteritis, osteomyelitis, arthritis
- *Campylobacter:* Guillain-Barré syndrome
- *Yersinia:* Erythema nodosum, erythema multiforme, reactive polyarthritis

Clostridium difficile

■ Epidemiology

- The most common identifiable pathogen in nosocomial diarrhea

■ TABLE 11-2   Antibiotic Recommendations for Specific Pathogens

Organism	Treatment
Aeromonas	Ciprofloxacin 500 mg twice daily for 3 days
Campylobacter	Azithromycin 500 mg twice daily for 3 days
EHEC	No treatment
Salmonella	Ciprofloxacin 500 mg twice daily for 5–7 days (treat only severe disease)
Shigella	Ciprofloxacin 500 mg twice daily for 3 days
Vibrio cholerae	Ciprofloxacin one dose of 1 g
Cryptosporidium	Nitazoxanide or paromomycin + azithromycin (severe disease or immunocompromised)
Cyclospora	TMP/SMX for 7 days
E. histolytica	Paromomycin for 7 days
Giardia	Metronidazole 250 mg three times daily for 5 days
Isospora	TMP/SMX twice daily for 10 days

Abbreviations: EHEC, enterohemorrhagic *E. coli*; TMP/SMX, trimethoprim-sulfamethoxazole

- **Risk factors:** Antibiotics, increased age, female gender (60% of cases), gastrointestinal manipulation (enemas, nasogastric tubes), inflammatory bowel disease, renal disease

■ Etiology
- Gram-positive anaerobic bacteria
- Two different toxins responsible for disease
  - **Toxin A:** Enterotoxin responsible for initial cellular damage and increased fluid accumulation in the bowel
  - **Toxin B:** Cytotoxin increases cellular damage through disruption of intracellular microfilaments, leading to cell rounding
- Infection can result in pseudomembranous colitis (PMC), antibiotic-associated colitis, or antibiotic-associated diarrhea

■ Pathogenesis
- Requires an alteration in normal gut flora allowing overgrowth of *C. difficile*
- Any antibiotic use, although clindamycin, ampicillin, and cephalosporins most commonly implicated

■ History
- Incubation period 1–10 days
- Asymptomatic

- Symptomatic: Loose bowel movements (90% to 95%), fever (80%), crampy abdominal pain (80% to 90%)

■ Additional Studies

- Imaging not routinely used. CT and barium enema can suggest PMC
- Endoscopy suggested for recurrent disease or diarrhea with negative toxin after antibiotic use
- Laboratory: Leukocytosis, leukopenia, thrombocytopenia, elevated C-reactive protein, elevated creatinine, hypokalemia, hypocalcemia, hypoalbuminemia, prolonged prothrombin time
- Fecal leukocytes: Less than 50% sensitivity (highly suggestive in right clinical scenario)
- ELISA: test for both toxins, very good sensitivity and specificity in animals

■ Differential Diagnosis

- Typhlitis (if neutropenic), ischemic colitis, inflammatory bowel disease, infectious colitis (*Campylobacter*, *Salmonella*, *Shigella*, *E. coli*)

■ Management

- Discontinue antibiotics if possible
- Oral **metronidazole** 250–500 mg four times daily for 7–14 days
- Oral **vancomycin** for 7–14 days if metronidazole contraindicated or not tolerated or severe disease
- Colestyramine for mild cases (although it binds vancomycin)
- Relapse or recurrence occur in 10% to 30% of cases
  - Retreat with metronidazole
  - Third episode: Use tapering or pulse-dose vancomycin
  - High-dose vancomycin in combination with either *Lactobacillus* GG or *Saccharomyces boulardii* demonstrates some success. "Fecal transplant" (rectal instillation of "normal" stool) is rarely used.
- **Surgical treatment:** Deterioration despite medical treatment

■ Complications

- Acute abdomen, sepsis, multiorgan failure, toxic dilation, perforation
- All of the above would prompt surgical evaluation

12 Genitourinary Tract Infections

Jeanne M. Marrazzo, MD, MPH

Urinary Tract Infections

- Includes asymptomatic bacteriuria, cystitis, prostatitis, pyelonephritis
- Cutoffs for significant bacteria counts in urine culture depend on circumstances (now $>10^2$/mL for young women)
- **Acute cystitis** common in young women; annual incidence 3% to 5%
- **Complicated urinary tract infections (UTIs)** more common with increasing age, male sex, nosocomial exposure

■ Risk Factors

- Acute cystitis in **young women:** Intercourse, prior UTI; Lewis blood group nonsecretor enhances *Escherichia coli* binding to target epithelial cells
- **Men:** Uncircumcised, incomplete micturition, insertive anal sex
- Pyelonephritis: **Pregnancy**
- **Complicated UTI** (involves stone or structural abnormality): Obstruction, vesicoureteral reflux, foreign body (kidney stone, catheter, tumor)

■ Etiology

- Acute cystitis/pyelonephritis/prostatitis: *E. coli* (75% to 90%); *Staphylococcus saprophyticus* (5% to 15%); *Klebsiella*, *Proteus* spp, enterococci, other (5% to 10%)
- Complicated UTI: Any of the above, especially *E. coli,* plus other gram-negative rods, *Staphylococcus aureus*, *Candida* spp

■ Pathogenesis

- Requires urethral colonization with bacteria; bladder entry facilitated by introital colonization/intercourse
- Certain *E. coli* strains are uropathogenic (bind avidly)
- Ascension of bacteria to cause pyelonephritis occurs in subset; hematogenous source is unusual
- Catheters provide biofilm matrix; facilitate bacterial growth, relatively impervious to antibiotic penetration

■ History

- **Cystitis:** Dysuria; urinary frequency, urgency; nocturia, suprapubic/back discomfort
- **Pyelonephritis:** Fever, rigors, flank pain, nausea, vomiting, cystitis symptoms
- **Prostatitis:** Fever, chills, perineal/back/pelvic pain, cystitis symptoms

■ Physical Examination

- **Cystitis:** Suprapubic tenderness
- **Pyelonephritis:** Costovertebral angle tenderness (often severe)
- **Prostatitis:** Tender, boggy prostate on digital rectal exam

■ Additional Studies

- Urinalysis: White blood cells (WBCs), leukocyte esterase, nitrite
- Gram stain of urine reveals bacteria
- Urine culture to determine bacterial etiology in all cases except uncomplicated acute cystitis (not necessary)
- More sophisticated imaging studies usually not necessary for pyelonephritis if patient responds rapidly to antibiotics; renal ultrasound if delay in response or other concerns
- Prostate-specific antigen (PSA) often elevated in acute prostates

■ Differential Diagnosis

- Pelvic inflammatory disease (PID) or other pelvic processes that cause localized pelvic tenderness
- Urethral infection with *Chlamydia trachomatis* or *Neisseria gonorrhoeae* (suspect if urinalysis shows inflammatory markers but no bacteria; patient may report recent new sex partner), or vulvovaginitis due to *Candida*, genital herpes
- Kidney stone (may be infected as well)

■ Management

- Cystitis
  - Healthy woman: Empiric 3 days oral trimethoprimsulfamethoxazole (TMP/SMX), fluoroquinolone (FQ; ciprofloxacin, levofloxacin, other), cefixime
  - Pregnancy: 7 days oral amoxicillin, nitrofurantoin preparation, cefixime, cefpodoxime
  - Male, diabetes, age over 65: Consider 7 days oral TMP/SMX, FQ (ciprofloxacin, levofloxacin, other), cefixime
- **Pyelonephritis:** 7 days oral ciprofloxacin if stable; parenteral therapy targeting gram-negative bacteria if required

- **Foley catheter:** Use clinical judgment; treat symptomatic UTI (fever, chills) with catheter removal, use of intermittent straight catheter or condom catheter during treatment. Sensitivities of responsible bacteria should be used to guide therapy
- **Asymptomatic bacteriuria:** Do not treat except in pregnancy

■ Complications

- Pregnancy: Pneumonia, adverse neonatal outcomes
- Acute papillary necrosis; emphysematous pyelonephritis (diabetics)
- Bacteremia, sepsis, renal abscess

Genital Skin/Mucosal Lesions

- Major groups include genital warts, caused by human papillomavirus (HPV) types 6/11; molluscum contagiosum; and genital ulcer disease (GUD), caused by herpes simplex virus (HSV); syphilis (both discussed in separate sections below); and chancroid
- Most sexually active adults infected with genital HPV at some point; minority develop warts
- Chancroid rare in US, associated with sex work
- Unprotected sex (risk: anal > vaginal > oral)

■ Etiology

- **Genital warts:** HPV-6/11
- **Chancroid:** *Haemophilus ducreyi*
- **Molluscum contagiosum:** Poxvirus

■ Pathogenesis

- Warts: Exuberant replication of HPV within epithelial cells
- Immunosuppression increases frequency/severity of warts and molluscum

■ History

- For genital warts/molluscum: Warty growths, painless bumps
- Chancroid ulcer often tender, may be multiple ulcers

■ Physical Examination

- **Warts:** Isolated verrucous lesions with cauliflower-like surface; often on shaft of penis or at vaginal introitus
- **Molluscum:** Small (1–2 mm) umbilicated papules with "pearl" expressed from center; usually genital area but may disseminate in immunocompromised

- **Chancroid:** Tender, ragged ulcer with purulent base
- Warts and molluscum are clinical diagnoses

■ Differential Diagnosis

- Pearly penile papules (normal variant), Tyson's glands (peri-urethral) can be mistaken for genital warts
- Fixed drug eruptions can ulcerate
- Systemic conditions including Behçet's syndrome
- For GUD, syphilis, and herpes (see below)

■ Management

- See **http://www.cdc.gov/std/treatment** for key updates
- Genital warts and molluscum eventually self-resolve in immunocompetent persons, but both can be treated with ablative therapy (cryotherapy [liquid nitrogen], podophyllin resin and toxin), and immunomodulators (imiquimod)
- Chancroid: Contact health department if suspected

Pelvic Inflammatory Disease and Cervicitis

- PID is inflammation of endometrium, Fallopian tubes, ovaries, or adnexa; perihepatitis (Fitz-Hugh-Curtis syndrome) and frank tubo-ovarian abscess (TOA) may occur
- Cervicitis defined as either easily induced bleeding or mucopurulent discharge from endocervical canal
- Both conditions caused by common STDs, especially *Chlamydia trachomatis* (CT) and *Neisseria gonorrhoeae* (GC) vaginal anaerobes important in PID
- Most CT and GC infections do not cause cervicitis, hence screening of women younger than 25 recommended annually; routine CT screening reduces rates of symptomatic PID
- Treating sex partners is critical
- Both cervicitis/PID most common in sexually active adolescents, parallel CT/GC epidemiology

■ Risk Factors

- **Unprotected intercourse** (no condoms), especially with new or multiple sex partners
- Cervical ectopy (site for CT/GC infection)
- Frequent **douching** (eradicates protective vaginal lactobacilli and erodes mucus plug)

■ Etiology

- Cervicitis: CT, GC; occasionally *Trichomonas vaginalis*, HSV (type 2 more common than type 1), *Mycoplasma genitalium*

- PID: CT, GC, vaginal bacteria; occasionally unusual bacteria (*Streptococcus pneumoniae, Actinomyces israeli*)

■ Pathogenesis

- CT/GC infect columnar epithelial cells of endocervix/ectropion
- Either/both ascend to upper genital tract, often accompanied by vaginal bacteria (predominantly anaerobes)

■ History

- Cervicitis: **Absent** (typical) or **nonspecific symptoms**—yellow-green vaginal discharge, intermenstrual bleeding
- PID: Lower abdominal/pelvic cramps or **dull pain;** Cervicitis symptoms

■ Physical Examination

- Cervicitis: Either easily induced bleeding or mucopurulent discharge from endocervical canal
- PID: Lower abdominal, uterine/adnexal, or cervical motion tenderness on bimanual exam. Specificity of diagnosis increased with Cervicitis or vaginal WBCs

■ Additional Studies

- Test all with Cervicitis/PID for CT and GC; evaluate vaginal fluid with pH, microscopy for bacterial vaginosis (BV), and trichomoniasis; herpes testing if suspected
- Moderate to severe PID: Consider transvaginal ultrasound if suspect TOA; peripheral complete blood count (CBC), erythrocyte sedimentation rate (ESR)
- Bacterial cultures of vaginal fluid not indicated

■ Differential Diagnosis

- PID: Any condition causing abdominal pain, including endometriosis, appendicitis, ovarian cyst rupture, midcycle pain, cholecystitis, gastroenteritis

■ Management

- See **http://www.cdc.gov/std/treatment** for key updates
- Cervicitis: Treat for CT given high prevalence; low threshold to treat for GC (young, sexually active)
  - CT: Azithromycin 1 g orally (PO) (single dose; preferred for compliance); doxycycline 100 mg PO twice daily for 7 days (avoid in pregnancy)
  - GC: Cefixime 400 mg PO (single-dose; if available); if FQ resistance not a problem, single-dose FQ (ciprofloxacin 500 mg PO, ofloxacin 400 mg PO)

- Mild-moderate PID: Requires **polymicrobial, multidose** outpatient antibiotics
  - Ceftriaxone 250 mg intramuscularly (IM) single-dose + doxycycline 100 mg PO twice daily for 14 days
  - Ofloxacin 400 mg PO twice daily or levofloxacin 500 mg PO daily + metronidazole 500 mg PO twice daily for 14 days
  - Return for assessment 24–48 hours
- Severe PID: Hospitalize for **parenteral therapy**
  - Clindamycin + gentamicin
  - Doxycycline plus either cefotetan or cefoxitin
  - Others: Ofloxacin or levofloxacin + metronidazole; ampicillin/sulbactam + doxycycline
- Treat all sex partners exposed in previous 60 days for CT/GC

■ Complications
- Untreated cervicitis can lead to PID
- Untreated PID major risk factor for tubal infertility, chronic pelvic pain, ectopic pregnancy

Urethritis

- ■ Male counterpart of cervicitis that typically represents STD (usually CT or GC)
- Most common among young men (under 25 y), parallels CT/GC trends
- Men who practice unprotected insertive anal sex: Urethritis caused by coliform bacteria (*E. coli*)

■ Etiology/Pathogenesis
- CT, GC most common; occasionally *Trichomonas vaginalis*, HSV, *Mycoplasma genitalium*, adenovirus
- Risk factors: Unprotected vaginal, anal, oral sex
- Infection of urethral columnar epithelial cells

■ History/ Physical Examination
- Dysuria, burning, urethral discharge
- Urethral discharge (purulent, serous, or seropurulent)

■ Additional Studies
- Gram stain of urethral discharge to quantify PMN (more than five PMN per high-power field is diagnostic), assess for gram-negative intracellular diplococci (98% sensitive for GC diagnosis)
- Test for CT/GC (highly sensitive nucleic acid amplification tests on first 15 mL of urine stream preferred, especially for CT)

■ **Differential Diagnosis**

- Occasionally can see allergic/irritant urethritis, but uncommon

■ **Management**

- See **http://www.cdc.gov/std/treatment** for key updates
- Treat for GC (see cervicitis section) if gram-positive; otherwise treat for CT unless coliforms likely (then treat with FQ)
- Evaluate/treat sex partners appropriately (exposed in last 60 days)

■ **Complications**

- Epididymitis, orchitis

Syphilis

- Syphilis can consist of **primary** (chancre), **secondary** (disseminated, often with rash, central nervous system [CNS] involvement), **tertiary** (gumma, tabes dorsalis, aortitis), or **latent** infection (serology-positive with no clinical disease)
- Divided into stages for management:
  - **Early:** Primary, secondary, early latent (less than 1 year)
  - **Late:** Late latent (1 year or more), tertiary
  - **Neurosyphilis:** Any CNS involvement
- Nearly eliminated in early 1990s in US, but reemerging in men who have sex with men (MSM)
- **Etiology:** Spirochete *Treponema pallidum;* cannot be cultured on artificial media

■ **Risk Factors**

- Unprotected vaginal, anal, oral sex or any contact to mucosal or skin lesions of secondary syphilis (highly infectious)
- Especially among MSM in urban centers, crystal methamphetamine users, anonymous partners arranged on Internet
- Birth to infected, untreated mother

■ **Pathogenesis**

- Untreated primary syphilis manifesting as GUD (chancre) resolves spontaneously, but *T. pallidum* returns in secondary form (disseminated disease) in ~30%
- Invasion of CNS can manifest as meningitis, cranial neuropathy, or latent disease (dementia, stroke)

■ **History**

- Chancre of syphilis **often painless,** but not reliable to use pain to distinguish *T. pallidum* as cause
- Report of unprotected sex with high-risk partner/situation

■ Physical Exam

- Primary: Chancre typically has clean base, is nontender; may occur anywhere on body, at site of inoculation, or in mouth
- Secondary: Diffuse rash often involving **palms/soles,** typically maculopapular but pustules or plaques can occur; condyloma lata (fleshy, wart-like growths in warm areas, typically perianal, scrotum, groin); **mucous patches** on tongue
- Tertiary: Very rare; bone, CNS gummas
- Neurosyphilis: Lymphocyte-predominant meningitis; uveitis; cranial nerve palsies (typically VII, VIII); mental status changes; tabes dorsalis (hyporeflexic wide-based gait)

■ Additional Studies

- Nontreponemal serology (RPR or VDRL) positive in 70% of primary, 99% of secondary, and 70% of tertiary and late latent; confirm with treponemal serology (TPPA or FTA-ABS)
- Primary syphilis: Darkfield microscopy of chancre exudate if available (requires experience)
- Cerebrospinal fluid (CSF) exam if any CNS signs/symptoms; consider increased protein or WBC, or a positive CSF VDRL to be consistent with CNS disease

■ Differential Diagnosis

- Any cause of GUD (herpes, chancroid)
- Any cause of rash (drug reaction, rickettsiosis, ehrlichiosis, pityriasis rosacea, tinea versicolor)

■ Management

- See **http://www.cdc.gov/std/treatment** for key updates
- **Early syphilis:** Benzathine penicillin 2.5 million units IM once (highly recommended); for severely penicillin-allergic, doxycycline 100 mg PO twice daily for 14 days
- **Late syphilis:** Benzathine penicillin 2.5 million units IM weekly for 3 weeks (highly recommended); for severely penicillin-allergic, doxycycline 100 mg PO twice daily for 28 days
- **Neurosyphilis:** Penicillin G intravenous (IV) 18–24 million units daily every 4 hours for 10–14 days; alternative is procaine penicillin 2.4 million units IM daily with probenecid 500 mg PO three times daily for 10–14 days
- Treat exposed partners (those from last 90 days)
- Follow quantitative nontreponemal serology to ensure response

■ Complications

- Severe neurologic, ophthalmic, orthopedic disease; high likelihood in untreated pregnant women of congenital syphilis causing severe congenital malformations, stillbirth, miscarriage

- **Jarisch-Herxheimer reaction:** Acute fever, headache, myalgia in first 24 hours after treatment; treat with nonsteroidal anti-inflammatory drug (NSAID)

Genital Herpes: HSV

- Among most common viral STD and most common cause of GUD worldwide
- Two main viruses: HSV-1 and HSV-2. HSV-2 causes most cases of recurrent genital herpes
- ~18% of persons older than 12 years in the US are seropositive for HSV-2
- Most (~80%) adults seropositive for HSV-1

■ Risk Factors

- Unprotected sex (risk: anal > vaginal > oral)
- Most genital herpes acquired from asymptomatic partners during periods of subclinical, unrecognized viral shedding

■ Etiology

- Genital herpes: HSV-2 in about 65% to 70%; remainder caused by HSV-1, typically through oral sex from partner with HSV-1 oral shedding (majority of adults seropositive for HSV-1)

■ Pathogenesis

- HSV ascends to dorsal root ganglia after primary infection to establish latency; reactivates with recurrences or subclinical shedding of virus from genital mucosa or affected skin
- Immunosuppression increases frequency/severity

■ History

- Initial herpes outbreak may be severe, especially women, with multiple vesicles (blisters), painful dysesthesias (burning), urinary retention, pelvic pain, meningeal or radicular signs
- Herpes recurrences tend to be less severe; prodrome common (tingling, pruritus at affected site)

■ Physical Examination

- Herpes classically **vesicles on erythematous base,** but after vesicle ruptures may resemble simple **eroded ulcer**
- May see erosive cervicitis, especially with primary HSV-2
- Subtle signs of recurrences include labial fissures, pruritic areas, often mistaken for vulvovaginal candidiasis, zipper injury

■ Additional Studies

- Often diagnosed by classic presentation, but recommend type-specific testing using culture or monoclonal antibody (direct fluorescent antibody [DFA]) to confirm initial diagnosis

- Accurate type-specific serology (glycoprotein Gg-based) now available

■ Differential Diagnosis

- Fixed drug eruptions can ulcerate
- Systemic conditions including Behçet's syndrome
- Other causes of GUD (syphilis, chancroid)

■ Management

- See **www.cdc.gov/std/treatment** for key updates
- Treat all initial episodes of genital herpes with 7–10 days PO of either acyclovir 400 mg three times daily; or valacyclovir 1 g twice daily; or famciclovir 250 mg three times daily
- Recurrent genital herpes: PO of either acyclovir 800 mg twice daily for 5 days; or valacyclovir 500 mg twice daily for 3–5 days or 1 g daily for 5 days (depending on severity); or famciclovir 125 mg twice daily for 5 days
- Suppressive oral therapy in persons with severe or frequent (four or more per year) recurrences: Acyclovir 400 mg twice daily OR valacyclovir 500 mg daily (nine or fewer annual recurrences) or 1 g daily; or famciclovir 250 mg twice daily. Reevaluate after ~1 year
- Suppressive therapy: Valacyclovir 500 mg PO daily reduces risk of transmission of HSV2 to susceptible sex partners by ~50%

■ Complications

- Genital herpes facilitates acquisition/transmission of HIV
- Acquisition of genital herpes in third trimester of pregnancy is major risk for neonatal herpes

13 Skin and Soft Tissue Infections

J. V. Hirschmann, MD

Streptococcal and Staphylococcal Skin Infections

- **Nasal carriage** of *Staphylococcus aureus* in normal population: **20% to 50% prevalence**
- 10% to 30% of people have never been nasal carriers of *S. aureus*; 20% to 30% are persistent carriers and 40% to 70% are intermittent carriers
- Increased risk of nasal carriage with insulin-dependent diabetes mellitus, injection drug abuse, hemodialysis, AIDS, eczema
- Most *S. aureus* skin infections are from patient's nasal flora
- Group A streptococcus (*Streptococcus pyogenes*) is not part of normal human flora. But transient carriage may occur, or organisms can survive for protracted periods on abnormal skin

■ Impetigo

Nonbullous Impetigo
- Most cases **caused by *S. aureus*.** But some are due to *S. pyogenes* or a combination of both organisms
- Most common in children, in summer, in warm/humid climates
- Often follows mild trauma, such as abrasions or insect bites
- Vesicles/pustules form with fragile roofs that rupture to form **honey-colored crusts**
- Impetigo heals without scarring

Bullous Impetigo
- Caused by *S. aureus* strains that produce epidermolytic toxin, causing a split in the epidermis, forming fragile blisters/pustules
- Bullous impetigo is more rare than nonbullous impetigo
- Pustules and blisters rupture to thin, brown, varnish-like crust
- Often the major findings are cutaneous erosions, with or without crusts, surrounded by a remnant of the blister's roof

■ Ecthyma
- Similar to nonbullous impetigo but infection is deeper affecting the dermis as well as epidermis, therefore leaving a scar
- Can be caused by *S. aureus* and/or *S. pyogenes*
- Often associated with poor hygiene, malnutrition, or alcoholism

- Typically on legs, although can be elsewhere; often follows minor trauma
- Pustules and vesicles become ulcers with thick, adherent crusts
- Culture and Gram stain can be obtained from material on the surface of the ulcer after removing the crust

■ Management of Impetigo and Ecthyma

- Topical mupirocin for 5–7 days for nonbullous impetigo
- Oral erythromycin, dicloxacillin, cephalexin for infections caused by *S. pyogenes* and methicillin-sensitive *S. aureus* (MSSA)
- For methicillin-resistant *S. aureus* (MRSA): topical mupirocin or oral treatment with clindamycin, trimethoprim-sulfamethoxazole (TMP/SMX), or doxycycline, depending on antimicrobial susceptibility

■ Other Staphylococcal Infections

Furuncle (Boil)

- Deep infection of hair follicle due to *S. aureus*
- Usually on head, neck, or arms
- Lesions are erythematous, tender nodules with central pustule through which hair emerges
- Management: Incision and drainage; antibiotics usually not needed
- Some patients—typically, nasal carriers of *S. aureus*—have recurrent attacks; prevention of recurrent attacks usually involves eradication of nasal carriage by either nasal mupirocin or oral clindamycin

Carbuncle

- Deep infection of adjacent hair follicles with *S. aureus*
- Patients commonly have diabetes
- Lesion is usually on back of neck, occasionally on back or thigh
- Painful, erythematous nodule with multiple sites of draining pus
- Management: Incision and drainage; antibiotics rarely indicated
- Area often heals slowly

Folliculitis

- A superficial inflammation of the hair follicle, causing erythematous papules and pustules
- With exposure to inadequately decontaminated **hot tubs, or swimming pools, the cause is often *Pseudomonas aeruginosa*,** which grows well in warm water
- Some contain normal skin flora, such as coagulase-negative staphylococci, *Corynebacterium* spp, and yeasts (*Malassezia furfur* or *Pityrosporum* spp)

- Many are sterile and presumably have noninfectious causes
- In adults, *S. aureus* is an uncommon cause

■ Pathogenesis

- *P. aeruginosa* proliferates in inadequately decontaminated water; organisms enter the hair follicle and cause inflammation
- In cases associated with normal skin flora or yeasts, the opening of the follicle probably becomes occluded by:
    - Excessive hydration (e.g., sweating) causing skin to swell
    - Friction from tight clothing causing excessive keratin formation
    - Excessive oiliness of the skin or oils from cosmetics
- Such occlusion traps organisms present on the surface of the skin in the follicle itself, provoking inflammation

■ History/Physical Exam

- In hot-tub folliculitis, itchy red papules appear on previously immersed portions of the body 8 hours to 5 days (mean 48 hours) after exposure
    - Lesions are 2–10 mm, often with central pinpoint pustule
    - Usual areas of involvement are buttocks, hips, arms, axillae, and thighs, with palms, soles, and mucous membranes unaffected
    - **Systemic complaints are rare,** but patients may have earaches
    - Resolves without therapy in a few days, usually does not scar
    - Other people who were in the water may also be affected, but attack rates among those exposed vary widely
- In other types of folliculitis, the trunk and thighs are most commonly affected by erythematous papules and pustules that may be itchy or occasionally painful

■ Additional Studies

- In hot-tub folliculitis, *P. aeruginosa* should grow from pus of a skin lesion and from the water in which the exposure occurred
- In other types of folliculitis, Gram stain of material from a pustule will demonstrate numerous neutrophils and:
    - Large, gram-positive oval structures, sometimes with budding, in types caused by yeasts
    - Gram-positive cocci and/or gram-positive bacilli in types due to normal skin bacteria

■ Management

- Hot-tub folliculitis is self-limited and requires no treatment, but the water in the tub needs to be decontaminated
- For folliculitis due to yeasts options include
    - Topical 2.5% selenium applied to affected areas
    - Ketoconazole shampoo or cream

- Oral fluconazole or itraconazole
- Recurrence is common; may repeat any of the above treatments
- For bacterial folliculitis, doxycycline for 1–2 weeks

Cutaneous Abscesses

- Collections of pus within the dermis and deeper tissues
- Most are **polymicrobial,** containing bacteria from local skin flora, often with organisms from an adjacent mucosal surface
- Abscesses of the head, neck, and trunk commonly grow coagulase-negative staphylococci and the anaerobic skin species *Propionibacterium* and *Peptostreptococcus*
- Abscesses of the genital/anal region commonly have fecal flora, including streptococci, *Bacteroides,* and other anaerobic bacteria
- *S. aureus,* usually alone, is present in ~25% to 50%
- Greater risk among injection drug users

■ Pathogenesis

- Minor trauma, often unnoticed, allows organisms to enter the dermis or deeper structures, causing neutrophilic inflammation

■ Physical Exam

- Painful, red, fluctuant nodules with variable surrounding erythematous edema, often with a pustule on top

■ Additional Studies

- No further studies usually needed. Gram stain/culture should be reserved for unusual infections or immunocompromised hosts

■ Management

- Incision with thorough evacuation of pus and probing the cavity to break up loculations
- Covering surgical site with dry dressing is usually adequate wound care, but some clinicians pack large wounds with gauze
- Local or systemic antibiotics are usually unnecessary, except for cutaneous gangrene, impaired host defenses, or severe systemic manifestations of infection (e.g., high fever)

Cellulitis

- Diffuse, spreading infection involving the dermis and subcutaneous fat

■ Risk Factors

- Preexisting edema from venous insufficiency, lymphedema, and other causes

- Previous skin damage, including surgery
- Maceration or scaling between toes, which allow colonization with streptococci that may invade the skin at that site or more proximally
- Breaks in the skin from trauma, cutaneous diseases such as eczema, or immersion injury

Etiology

- Cultures of needle aspiration and skin biopsies are usually negative, indicating low numbers of organisms present
- Most cases are caused by streptococci, not only group A, but also other groups such as C or G
- Streptococci are often present in toe web skin abnormalities, which serve as a reservoir in patients with recurrent episodes
- *S. aureus* can cause cellulitis, but is usually associated with an open wound or an abscess. *Pasteurella* **species often cause cellulitis following injury from a dog or cat**
- Cellulitis following exposure to warm salt water can be from *Vibrio vulnificus*, and following immersion in fresh water can be from *Aeromonas hydrophila*, both gram-negative bacilli
- In **neutropenic patients,** gram-negative bacilli, such as *Pseudomonas aeruginosa,* can cause cellulitis
- In patients with severe **cell-mediated immune deficiency,** *Cryptococcus neoformans* can be a cause

Pathogenesis

- Organisms and their toxins elicit inflammation in the dermis and subcutaneous fat, causing cutaneous erythema and edema
- The inflammation can affect the lymphatic system, causing lymphangitis, which is visible as linear erythema on the skin. Some damage to the lymphatics occurs with each episode, and chronic lymphedema may develop with repeated attacks

History/Physical Exam

- Patients can have fevers and chills develop even before skin changes, but many patients are afebrile
- The most common sites are the legs. Other frequent areas of cellulitis include arms, abdomen, and face
- Involved skin demonstrates diffuse redness, heat, edema, and tenderness. The surface appearance may resemble an orange skin (peau d'orange), with dimpling at the site of hair follicles
- **Red streaks, representing lymphangitis,** may extend proximally, and regional lymph nodes may be warm, enlarged, and tender

Additional Studies

- The white blood cell count may be elevated and/or have increased bands, but it may be completely normal

- **Blood cultures are positive in fewer than 5% of cases,** but may be worthwhile in very ill patients or those with unusual exposures (such as immersion injuries), immunodeficiency, or neutropenia
- Needle aspiration of involved skin provides a positive culture in about 5%, but yield is higher if there is an abscess or necrotic skin
- Skin punch biopsies are culture-positive in about 20%, but are not usually indicated except in immunocompromised patients

■ Management

- Antibiotic therapy directed against streptococci. Many also treat *S. aureus*. Dicloxacillin or cephalexin often used for oral treatment. If patient has severe penicillin allergy, clindamycin is reasonable. For patients too ill for oral therapy, IV oxacillin or nafcillin, cefazolin, or clindamycin are good choices
- For cellulitis following animal bites, see next section for antibiotic choices. For suspected *V. vulnificus* infection from salt-water injury or *A. hydrophila* from fresh-water exposure, a fluoroquinolone, or a third-generation cephalosporin is reasonable
- Elevation of the affected area is important to help resolve edema and allow toxic products to drain into the circulation by gravity
- Oral corticosteroids may help the cellulitis resolve more quickly and may reduce lymphangitis and long-term lymphedema
- Cellulitis and the systemic manifestations, such as fever, may worsen following treatment, probably due to abrupt killing of organisms and the release of toxins exacerbating inflammation
- Patients with leg cellulitis should be treated for toe-web abnormalities and associated fungal infection or erythrasma (a common interdigital infection caused by *Corynebacterium* spp) to help eliminate the reservoir of organisms that may cause recurrence. An azole antifungal, such as miconazole or clotrimazole, is effective against erythrasma or fungal infections
- Patients with numerous episodes despite attempts to control edema, interdigital abnormalities, and other reversible problems may benefit from prophylactic antibiotics. Good options are penicillin, erythromycin, or benzathine penicillin

Infected Animal Bites

- During their lifetime, about half of Americans will be bitten by an animal, by a dog more often than a cat. The animal is usually known to the victims, about 20% of whom seek medical advice

- About 15% of dog bites and 60% of cat bites become infected
- The risk of infection is greatest for crush injuries, punctures, and hand wounds

■ Etiology

- The **average infected wound yields five types of bacteria,** with ~60% yielding mixed aerobic and anaerobic organisms and 40% aerobic organisms alone. Predominant pathogens are normal oral flora of the biting animal, combined with some human skin flora and secondary invaders such as *S. pyogenes* and *S. aureus*
- *Pasteurella* species are isolated from 50% of dog bites and 75% of cat bites
- Staphylococci and streptococci occur in about 40% of infected wounds
- Anaerobes are present in 65% of cat bites and 50% of dog bites

■ History/Physical Exam

- Bite infections appear as cellulitis, purulent wounds, or abscesses. Fever, inflamed regional lymph nodes, and lymphangitis may be present
- Signs of infection appear ~12 hours after cat bites, ~24 hours after dog bites. *Pasteurella* **infections develop and progress rapidly**
- Physical exam should be thorough and the clinician should document a diagram of the location, extent of the injuries, range of motion of the area, and any evidence of tendon or nerve injuries or extension to bone or joint

■ Management

Clinically Infected Bite Wounds

- Clinicians should rinse the wound with sterile normal saline and remove superficial debris. Abscesses should be incised and drained. Cultures of purulent material should be obtained
- Patient should receive **tetanus toxoid** if more than 5 years since last dose
- Elevation of injury hastens resolution of inflammatory edema
- Appropriate oral antibiotic therapy for infected bites includes **amoxicillin-clavulanate** or, for penicillin-allergic patients, doxycycline. Cellulitis and purulent wounds usually respond to 5–10 days of treatment

Early, Clinically Uninfected Bite Wounds

- Patients with uninfected wounds less than 12 hours old should have saline irrigation and tetanus prophylaxis
- The closure of early wounds is debated. A reasonable approach is to approximate the wound edges with adhesive strips and

allow closure by secondary intent or perform delayed primary closure. Facial wounds, however, can be closed primarily
- Antibiotic therapy for early wounds is controversial, but may be appropriate for those that are moderate to severe, adjacent to bone or joint, have crush injury or edema, affect the hands, or are facial injuries that have received primary closure. Amoxicillin-clavulanate or doxycycline for 3–5 days should suffice

Infected Human Bites

- Human bites are the third most common bites, behind dogs and cats. They are often more serious and prone to infection
- Human bites may be occlusive wounds, in which the teeth actually bite the body part, or clenched-fist wounds, in which the hand strikes the teeth
- Most human bites occur during altercations, but some occlusive wounds are "love nips" related to sexual activity

■ Etiology

- Primarily bacteria from the oral flora of the biter
- The median number of organisms cultured from these wounds is four, about three aerobes and one anaerobe. The major aerobic isolates are **oral streptococci, _S. aureus,_ and _Eikenella corrodens,_** a gram-negative coccobacillus. The major anaerobes are _Prevotella_ and _Fusobacterium_ spp, both gram-negative bacilli, and _Veillonella_ spp, which are gram-negative cocci

■ History/Physical Exam

- Infected human bite findings are abscesses, purulent wounds, or nonpurulent wounds with cellulitis and/or lymphangitis
- The median time from injury to appearance of infection is about 22 hours, but with **cellulitis or lymphangitis** it is 6 hours

■ Management

Clinically Infected Human Bites
- Many patients require hospital admission and **IV antibiotics**
- Abscesses need drainage
- A hand care expert should evaluate patients with clenched fist injuries to determine if there has been penetration into bone, joint capsule, or synovium. Surgical exploration may be necessary
- Elevate injury to reduce edema. With hand wounds, splinting in a position of function reduces later stiffness
- For **outpatient oral antimicrobial therapy,** amoxicillin-clavulanate is a good choice; for penicillin-allergic patients, a fluoroquinolone, such as levofloxacin, plus clindamycin or a

combination of TMP/SMX and metronidazole should be effective

- For IV therapy, appropriate alternatives include ampicillin-sulbactam or cefotetan; with penicillin or cephalosporin allergy, clindamycin plus a fluoroquinolone is reasonable
- Duration of therapy depends on clinical findings and treatment response, but 1–2 weeks is often adequate. For septic arthritis or osteomyelitis, most patients are treated for 4–6 weeks

Early, Clinically Uninfected Human Bites

- As with animal bites, irrigation and topical wound cleansing
- Because of the high risk of infection, antimicrobial therapy of early wounds that show no signs of inflammation is reasonable, using the oral medications mentioned above for 3–5 days

Necrotizing Fasciitis

A severe soft tissue infection with necrosis of the fascia and sub-cutaneous tissue. Involvement of the genitalia is called Fournier's gangrene, named after a nineteenth-century French clinician

■ Risk Factors

- Most patients have underlying disorder that affects local or sys-temic host defenses, such as diabetes mellitus, alcoholism, AIDS, illicit drug use, or peripheral vascular disease
- Patients often have area of **skin damage,** such as a cut, abrasion, burn, injection, or surgical incision through which infecting organisms have entered. The trauma may be minor, such as an insect bite. In ~15%, no preceding injury is apparent

■ Etiology

- A few infections are due to a single organism, usually *S. pyogenes* (group A streptococcus) or, less often, *V. vulnificus*, a marine bacterium, from exposure to salt water, fish, or crustaceans
- Most infections are **polymicrobial,** with an average of about five different organisms isolated, typically a combination of two types of aerobic and three types of anaerobic bacteria. The most common aerobic isolates are various streptococci, *S. aureus*, and enteric gram-negative bacilli such as *E. coli* and *Klebsiella* spp. The most common anaerobes are *Peptostreptococcus*, *Bacteroides*, and *Clostridium* spp

■ Pathogenesis

- A skin break allows organisms into the subcutaneous space, where they cause tissue inflammation and thrombosis of the microvasculature, leading to necrosis. Gas may form from

hydrogen and nitrogen (the products of anaerobic metabolism by enteric gram-negative bacilli and strictly anaerobic bacteria)
- The muscle underlying the deep fascia is usually unaffected, but compromised circulation to the overlying skin can cause cutaneous edema, erythema, hemorrhage, blister formation, and, eventually, gangrene
- Damage to fascia decreases its adherence to adjacent structures, allowing **infection to spread laterally along tissue planes**

■ History/Physical Exam

- In those with an identifiable injury, clinical features usually begin within a few days of the event
- Major features are erythema, heat, swelling, and tenderness, most often of the extremities, but possibly affecting any body region. The **edema characteristically extends beyond the erythema,** helping distinguish this from uncomplicated cellulitis
- Pain is typically much worse than physical findings suggest. Most patients are febrile. Many appear "toxic," with flushing, sweating, and listlessness, sometimes with hypotension
- As the disease progresses, cutaneous hemorrhage, bullae, gangrene, and crepitus may develop. Damage to the cutaneous nerves can render **some skin areas anesthetic**
- When group A streptococci are present, **streptococcal toxic shock syndrome** can occur, with hypotension, generalized erythematous macular rash that may desquamate, and multiorgan involvement (renal impairment, abnormal liver tests, thrombocytopenia, and acute respiratory distress syndrome)

■ Additional Studies

- Patients typically have a neutrophilic leukocytosis. Blood cultures are worthwhile, but are typically negative with polymicrobial infections; they are more commonly positive when *S. pyogenes* or *V. vulnificus* are causes
- Plain films may show **subcutaneous gas.** Computed tomography (CT) or magnetic resonance imaging (MRI) scans may reveal fluid collections, but often these studies are unnecessary
- Needle aspiration may yield pus, which can be sent for Gram stain/culture, as should any material obtained at surgery

■ Differential Diagnosis

- The major distinction is from uncomplicated cellulitis. Lymphangitis and inflamed regional lymph nodes are rare in necrotizing fasciitis but may be present in cellulitis
- Features strongly suggesting necrotizing fasciitis are:
  - **Pain disproportionately severe compared to physical findings**
  - Cutaneous bullae, hemorrhage, gangrene, or rapid spread

    - Edema extending beyond the erythema
    - **Crepitus** or gas in tissue on imaging studies

■ Management

- The major therapy is **surgical debridement.** The findings are typically necrosis of the superficial fascia and fat, and thick or thin pus, which is commonly foul-smelling when anaerobes are present

- The goal of surgery is to remove pus and necrotic tissue. May require **several operations, often scheduled at 24-hour intervals** until no further necrotic material is present

- During the operation, a blunt probe or finger typically extends readily in a plane between fascia and dermis, which are ordinarily tightly connected. The surgeon should continue the incision until such a maneuver is no longer possible

- Patient should receive empiric IV antibiotics potent against streptococci, enteric gram-negative bacilli, and anaerobic bacteria. Ampicillin-sulbactam should suffice for community-acquired infections, although vancomycin should be added for drug abusers and other situations in which MRSA infections are likely. Cefotetan or a combination of gentamicin and clindamycin are reasonable alternatives. Clindamycin is recommended in suspected streptococcal toxic shock syndrome to decrease toxin production from the bacteria

- For **nosocomial infections,** piperacillin-tazobactam, imipenem or meropenem, or a combination of ceftazidime and clindamycin are reasonable choices among many options

■ Complications

- To control infection and remove all necrotic tissue, some patients require amputation of an extremity. Others are left with substantial wounds that require later skin grafts

- The overall mortality rate is about 20% to 30%, with delay in obtaining surgery substantially increasing the risk of death

14 Bone and Joint Infections

Ahmet C. Tural, MD

Septic Arthritis

Inflammation of the joint space due to infection

■ Pathogenesis
- Hematogenous inoculation
- Direct extension from adjacent bone infection
- Trauma, surgery, intra-articular injection

■ Risk Factors
- Preexisting arthritis: Rheumatoid arthritis, osteoarthritis, gout, Charcot's arthropathy
- Trauma
- Underlying immunocompromised state: HIV, malignancy, diabetes mellitus, hypogammaglobulinemia
- Age over 60 years
- **Intravenous drug users (IVDU)**
- Indwelling catheters

■ Etiology
- Acute bacterial arthritis
  - *Staphylococcus aureus:* Most common
  - *Streptococcus pyogenes*, other streptococcal spp
  - Gram-negative bacilli: 10% to 20% of cases; more common in IVDU, immunodeficient hosts, elderly
  - *Neisseria gonorrhoeae:* Women during **menstrual cycle** or pregnancy
  - *Haemophilus influenzae*, type b: Rare since introduction of conjugate vaccine
  - *Borrelia bungdorferi*
  - Anaerobes: Rare
  - **10% of cases are polymicrobial**
- Mycobacterial arthritis
  - *Mycobacterium tuberculosis*
  - Atypical mycobacteria
    - *M. kansasii, M. marinum, M. fortuitum*

- Fungal arthritis
  - *Coccidioides immitis, Sporothrix schenckii, Cryptococcus neoformans, Candida* spp
- Viral arthritis
  - Rubella, mumps, hepatitis B, parvovirus, enteroviruses

■ History

- Bacterial arthritis: Most present acutely with **fever, and a swollen, painful joint**

■ Physical Exam

- Joint effusion, tenderness, limited range of motion
- Skin lesions and tenosynovitis with disseminated gonococcal infection
- **Septic bursitis** (olecranon, prepatellar) following local trauma

■ Additional Studies

Lab Tests

- Peripheral leukocytosis, elevated erythrocyte sedimentation rate (ESR); **blood cultures are positive in ~50% of bacterial arthritis**
- Synovial fluid analysis
  - Bacterial: Turbid, white blood cells **(WBCs) usually over 50,000/mm^3** (with over 75% neutrophils), glucose less than 40 mg/dL or less than half of serum level, bacteria on smears in ~30%, culture growth in ~90%
  - Viral: Modest elevation of WBC (mostly monocytes)
  - Polymerase chain reaction (PCR): Available for Lyme and gonococcal arthritis

Imaging Studies

- Perform x-ray and ultrasound; magnetic resonance imaging (MRI) not routinely required
- X-rays usually normal; may reveal **capsular swelling,** fat pad displacement, and adjacent soft tissue swelling. Later in course, detects joint space narrowing due to cartilage destruction. Most important to exclude other causes such as fracture
- Ultrasound: Detects effusion and guides arthrocentesis
- MRI: Detects joint effusion and associated soft tissue swelling or osteomyelitis

■ Differential Diagnosis

- Crystal-induced arthritis: History, crystals in synovial fluid
- Systemic rheumatic diseases
- Reactive, traumatic
- Hemarthrosis

■ Management

- Initial antimicrobials based on Gram stain results:
  - Gram-positive cocci: Cefazolin for community-acquired (use vancomycin in areas with high methicillin-resistant *S. aureus* [MRSA] prevalence), vancomycin for nosocomial infection
  - Gram-negative bacilli: Ceftriaxone or, if *Pseudomonas* likely, ceftazidime + gentamicin
  - Negative Gram stain: Cefazolin
  - Modify antimicrobials according to culture results
- Duration of therapy: Usually **4 weeks** (at least 14 days parenteral)
- **Joint drainage**
  - Hip, shoulder, weight-bearing joints, persistent effusion for more than 7 days: Surgical drainage
  - Other joints: Needle aspiration (repeat as needed)
- Avoid weight bearing. Immobilization not necessary

■ Complications

- Limitation of joint motion, amputation, arthrodesis, prosthetic surgery, persistent pain

Osteomyelitis

Infection resulting in inflammatory destruction of the bone
- Acute: Evolves over **days to weeks**
- Chronic: Long-standing infection that evolves (arbitrarily) over **months to years**

■ Pathogenesis

- Three mechanisms of acquisition: (1) **Hematogenous,** (2) contiguous-focus (e.g., direct spread from a contiguous focus of infection or from a penetrating wound), and (3) vascular insufficiency-related (e.g., diabetic patients)
- Bone destruction results from several mechanisms
  - Compression/destruction of vascular channels causes bone ischemia followed by necrosis
  - Osteoclastic activity at edge of necrotic area causes additional bone loss and localized osteoporosis
  - Invading bacteria produce **exotoxins or hydrolases** that degrade host cells or extracellular matrix, respectively
- **Necrotic bone** impedes successful treatment, because the bone may still harbor bacteria, but the lack of blood supply isolates them from antibiotics and host immune response

■ Risk Factors

- Trauma
- Large organism inoculation
- Presence of foreign body
- Neuropathy

■ Etiology

- Hematogenous: *S. aureus* most common (almost always single infecting organism)
- Contiguous-focus (e.g., penetrating trauma) and vascular insufficiency-related: *S. aureus*, polymicrobial aerobic gram-negative bacilli, anaerobes
- Special considerations
  - Vertebral osteomyelitis: *S. aureus*, **P. aeruginosa** (in IVDU), *E. coli*, *Klebsiella* spp, *M. tuberculosis*
  - Prosthetic joint: **Coagulase-negative staphylococci**, *S. aureus*, *E. coli*, *Klebsiella* spp, *Streptococcus* spp
  - Immunocompromised patients: Also consider *Candida* spp, *Aspergillus* spp, and *M. tuberculosis*

■ History

- Preceding bacteremic illness
- Recent trauma, surgery, soft tissue infection

■ Physical Exam

- Nonspecific pain, constitutional symptoms, sometimes fevers, chills, localized erythema, swelling, tenderness

■ Additional Studies

- Initial lab studies
  - Blood cultures: More likely positive in acute rather than chronic osteomyelitis
  - ESR, C-reactive protein (CRP), peripheral WBC: Often elevated but not diagnostic
- Radiologic evaluation
  - Plain films: **Not sensitive or specific**
    - Acute: Soft tissue swelling or periosteal reaction in early phase. Bone destruction not visible until after 10 days of infection.
    - Chronic: Bone sclerosis, periosteal new bone formation, sequestra (separated necrotic bone segment devoid of blood supply)
  - Computed tomography (CT): **Cortical destruction,** intra-osseous gas, periosteal reaction, surrounding soft tissue changes

- Radionuclide studies: Three-phase bone scan, indium-labeled leukocyte scan. Useful for whole-body examinations
- MRI: Especially useful in evaluating foot and vertebrae. **More sensitive** than radionuclide studies
- Cultures taken at bone biopsy or debridement surgery
  - **Biopsy mandatory in chronic osteomyelitis** or if symptoms minimally improved after 5–7 days of antibiotic therapy
  - Send aerobic, anaerobic, mycobacterial, and fungal cultures; Gram stain; and histopathology
  - More than 5 neutrophils per high-power field suggests bacterial infection with sensitivity of 40% to 60% and specificity of over 90%
  - **Granulomatous lesions** (by histopathology) suggest **mycobacteria**

■ Management

- Antimicrobials
  - Usually requires **6 weeks** of parenteral treatment
  - Shorter course of parenteral therapy, followed by oral (PO) therapy acceptable (e.g., 2 weeks parenteral + 4–6 weeks PO)
  - Empiric therapy directed to most likely pathogen(s)
    - *Staphylococcus aureus:* Nafcillin or cefazolin, add rifampin in prosthetic joint infections
    - MRSA: Vancomycin + rifampin; linezolid also effective but costly
    - Beta-hemolytic streptococci: Clindamycin
    - Enteric gram-negative bacilli: Fluoroquinolone or cefotaxime
    - *Pseudomonas aeruginosa:* Ceftazidime + aminoglycoside
    - Mixed (aerobic and anaerobic) infection: Ampicillin-sulbactam or ticarcillin-clavulanate or imipenem
- **Surgical therapy:** Often indicated in adults
  - Failure to respond to antimicrobial therapy
  - Presence of abscess
  - Concomitant joint infection

■ Complications

- Chronic or recurrent osteomyelitis
- Osteoporosis, disuse atrophy
- Limb loss

15 Bloodstream Infections

Caroline B. Long, MD and Samir S. Shah, MD

Sepsis

■ Epidemiology

- Clinical syndrome defined by presence of both bloodstream infection (BSI) and dysregulated systemic inflammatory response
- More than 650,000 cases of sepsis and 100,000 sepsis-related deaths annually
- Accounts for over 8% of intensive care unit (ICU) admissions

■ Risk Factors

- Bloodstream or urinary tract infection
- Age under 1 year or over 55 years
- Comorbidities depressing host defenses (e.g., neoplasm, AIDS)
- Prolonged central catheter use and extended ICU stay

■ Etiology

- Gram-positive bacteria: Coagulase-negative *Staphylococcus* and *Staphylococcus aureus* account for over 50% of cases
- Gram-negative bacteria (especially *Escherichia coli*, *Klebsiella pneumoniae*, *Enterobacter* spp)
- Others: Fungal (5%), polymicrobial (5%),anaerobes (2%), occasionally *Candida* spp or *Rickettsia* spp

■ Pathogenesis

- Combination of direct pathogen effect (e.g., via endotoxin) and dysregulated host response (via cytokines such as tumor necrosis factor-alpha and interleukin-1) lead to cellular ischemia, cytopathic injury, and apoptosis

■ History/Physical Exam

- Hypotension (systolic less than 90 mm Hg; mean arterial pressure [MAP] less than 60 mm Hg, or more than 40 mm Hg below baseline MAP)
- Tachycardia (more than 90 bpm)
- Hyper- or hypothermia (temperature over 100.4°F [38°C] or under 96.8°F [36°C])

- Altered mental status
- Chills, petechiae, purpura, and cyanosis
- Organ failure (e.g., oliguria, anuria, jaundice)

■ Additional Studies

- Two peripheral blood cultures
- Complete blood count to evaluate for leukocytosis or leukopenia, left shift (bandemia, neutrophil predominance), and thrombocytopenia
- Basic metabolic panel to evaluate for acidosis and renal dysfunction
- Evaluate for **coagulopathy:** Increased prothrombin/partial thromboplastin time (PT/PTT), increased d-dimers, increased fibrin split products, decreased fibrinogen
- Arterial blood gas (**acidosis or hypoxemia**)
- Other tests to **identify source of infection** as directed by history and exam (e.g., urine culture, abdominal computed tomography [CT], ultrasound)

■ Differential Diagnosis

- Noninfectious activation of systemic inflammatory response (pancreatitis, severe burn, multiple traumatic injury), anaphylaxis, drug or toxin reaction (including insect bite and transfusion reaction), Addisonian crisis

■ Management

- Empiric **broad-spectrum** combination antimicrobial therapy allows: (1) Coverage for a wide range of bacteria that may be difficult to distinguish clinically; (2) **potential synergy** between two antimicrobials to enhance the sum of antimicrobial activity; and (3) coverage for the possibility of **polymicrobial** bacteremia
- Empiric regimens are specific to presumed etiology:
  - Life-threatening infection, unknown source: Imipenem or meropenem. Alternative regimen: Aminoglycoside (e.g., gentamicin, amikacin) + one of the following: third- or fourth-generation cephalosporin, piperacillin-tazobactam, or ticarcillin-clavulanate
  - Community acquired, suspected urinary tract source: Third-generation cephalosporin + aminoglycoside, or fluoroquinolone (e.g., ciprofloxacin, gatifloxacin)
  - Community acquired, suspected nonurinary tract source: Third-generation cephalosporin + metronidazole; ticarcillin-clavulanate, piperacillin-tazobactam, or ampicillin-sulbactam ± aminoglycoside

- Hospital acquired infection: Cefepime + aminoglycoside ±
  metronidazole
- In areas of high methicillin-resistant *S. aureus* (MRSA)
  prevalence or if central venous catheter (CVC) present, consider adding vancomycin
- Modify regimen based on culture results and sensitivity patterns
- Drotrecogin alfa (**activated protein C,** also called Xigris); 60%
  to 90% of septic patients have low activated protein C levels.
  PROWESS study showed a decrease in 28-day mortality from
  30.8% to 24.7% with use of Xigris in acutely ill patients. Major
  adverse effect is **bleeding** in 0.4% to 3.5% of patients receiving
  Xigris versus 0.2% to 2.0% receiving placebo. Treatment typically given continuously for 72 hours (daily cost $1500 to
  $2000). According to PROWESS study, one patient is saved for
  every 16 receiving treatment
- Corticosteroid therapy improves 28-day mortality only in a
  subgroup of patients with septic shock or sepsis-induced organ
  dysfunction who were unresponsive to adrenocorticotropic
  hormone (ACTH) stimulation challenge test
- Rigorous control of blood glucose improves outcome

■ Complications

- Severe sepsis: Sepsis with multiorgan dysfunction secondary to
  hypoperfusion and direct cellular injury (most common cause
  of death in noncardiac intensive care unit [ICU])
- Septic shock: Acute circulatory failure with persistent arterial
  hypotension despite adequate volume resuscitation (more
  common in sepsis due to gram-negative bacilli)
- Multiple organ dysfunction syndrome (MODS): Most severe
  end of spectrum of severity of illness. Common manifestations
  include acute respiratory distress syndrome (ARDS), acute
  renal failure, and disseminated intravascular coagulation (DIC)
- Mortality approximately 40% for all kinds of sepsis but varies
  by organism
- Mortality higher in nosocomial-acquired BSI

Central Venous Catheter-Related Infection

■ Epidemiology

- CVC-related infection may be local (e.g., insertion site cellulitis)
  or systemic (BSI)
- More than 5 million CVCs inserted annually
- 90% of nosocomial BSIs are CVC-related
- More than 175,000 CVC-related BSIs annually

■ TABLE 15-1	Types of Central Venous Catheters
Nontunneled	Subclavian, internal jugular, or femoral single-, double-, or triple-lumen device inserted centrally
	Swan-Ganz catheter
	Peripherally inserted central catheter (PICC)
Tunneled (surgically inserted)	Hickman
	Broviac
	Groshong
	Quinton
Totally implantable intravascular device	Portacath
	Hemodialysis catheter (Perma-cath)

- CVC-related BSI prolongs hospitalization by a mean of 7 days and increases medical costs by over $6000

■ **Risk Factors**

- Intrinsic factors: Extremes of age, underlying illness, malnutrition, loss of skin integrity (e.g., **burns**)
- Extrinsic factors: Catheter location, duration of catheterization, type of device, conditions of insertion, site care, skill of inserter
- 90% of catheter-related BSI are secondary to nontunneled CVCs (Table 15-1)
- Higher risk with (1) internal jugular CVC; (2) nontunneled > tunneled > totally implanted device
- Lower risk with (1) silver chelated collagen cuff; (2) antimicrobial drug-impregnated catheters (e.g., minocycline + rifampin, chlorhexidine + silver sulfadiazine); (3) chlorhexidine prep compared to Betadine prep
- Exchanging over guide wire at routine intervals does not decrease risk

■ **Etiology**

- Gram-positive cocci (coagulase-negative *Staphylococcus* and *S. aureus*) are most common pathogens
- Gram-negative bacilli (30% cases)
- Fungi (20% of cases; increased risk for fungal infection in patients receiving high concentration of glucose via intravenous hyperalimentation)

■ **Pathogenesis**

- Four major sources: (1) Colonization of skin (most common); (2) catheter lumen or hub contamination; (3) secondary seeding of catheter from BSI (most likely in critically ill patient);

and (4) rarely, contamination of infusate (can cause epidemic infection)
- Biofilm on catheter lumen is important in colonization process (derived from a combination of host and microbe products) and produces a nidus for infection

■ History/Physical Exam

- Clinical findings are similar to those described for sepsis
- More specific signs include: Inflammation or purulence at insertion site, dysfunction of catheter, clinical signs of sepsis that start abruptly after infusion, rapid improvement upon CVC removal

■ Additional Studies

- Simultaneous CVC and peripheral blood cultures to determine whether catheter is the source of infection
  - Quantitative blood cultures: Findings that suggest CVC as the source of infection include (1) CVC culture yields a **colony count by quantitative culture at least 5-fold higher than peripheral blood culture;** (2) 15 or more colony-forming units (CFUs) from catheter tip by **semiquantitative culture** (colony counts directly from agar plate); (3) 100 or more CFUs from catheter tip by **quantitative culture** (serial dilutions of original specimen allows for more precise enumeration of colony count)
  - Alternative (easier) method is differential time to positivity: Positive result from CVC culture at least 2 hours earlier than from peripheral culture. Compared to quantitative blood culture methods, **differential time to positivity** has sensitivity of 80% to 90% and specificity of 75% to 94%
- Culture and Gram stain of exudate from infected insertion site
- **Transesophageal echocardiogram** in all patients (unless contraindicated) with catheter-related *S. aureus* BSI to look for complicating endocarditis
- Additional laboratory evaluation similar to that for sepsis

■ Management

Empiric Therapy

- Therapy determined by nature and severity of infection, type of device, method of insertion (e.g., tunneled), infecting pathogen, underlying host status, presence or absence of alternative venous access site, and anticipated duration of therapy
- Empiric antibiotic regimen consists of vancomycin plus an aminoglycoside (e.g., gentamicin or tobramycin). Linezolid is appropriate alternative for patients at high risk for infection with vancomycin-resistant enterococci

TABLE 15-2 Catheter Management in Patients with CVC-Related Infection

Type of Infection	Catheter Management
Local Infection	
Insertion site[a]	Remove CVC (don't change over guide wire because of risk of septic emboli)
Exit site	Remove CVC if:
	No longer required
	Alternative site exists
	Patient clinically septic
	Infection due to *Pseudomonas* or fungi
Tunneled/Pocket	Remove CVC
Systemic Infection	Remove CVC if:
	S. aureus, gram-negative rods, polymicrobial, or fungal
	Failure to respond clinically
	Failure to clear bacteremia in 48–72 hours
	Insertion site infection
	Septic appearance
	Granulocytopenia
	Noninfectious valvular heart disease (increased risk of endocarditis)
	Endocarditis
	Metastatic abscesses
	Septic thrombophlebitis

[a] With PICC, the exit and insertion sites are the same; with surgically implanted and tunneled catheters, the original insertion site is closed and a separate exit site is created

- Modify regimen based on clinical response, culture results, and susceptibility patterns
- See Table 15-2 for catheter removal recommendations

Duration of Therapy
- Local infection
  - If blood cultures are negative, treat for 7 days
  - If patient does not meet criteria for immediate removal of catheter (Table 15-2), treatment without removal is successful in more than 50% of exit site infections

- Systemic infection
  - **Repeat blood cultures** until a negative culture is documented (to demonstrate clearance of BSI)
  - Coagulase-negative *Staphylococcus*: Treat for 5–7 days if CVC removed, 10–14 days if CVC retained
  - *S. aureus*: Treat for 14 days. If transesophageal echocardiogram positive, extend treatment to 4–6 weeks for endocarditis
  - *Candida* spp: Treat for 14 days after last positive blood culture
  - Gram-negative bacilli: Treat for 10–14 days
  - Longer duration of therapy if: (1) failure to respond clinically, (2) failure to clear BSI within 48–72 hours, (3) immunocompromised host, (4) preexisting valvular heart disease, and (5) complicating endocarditis or osteomyelitis
- Possible benefit of **antibiotic-lock therapy** (filling catheter lumen with antibiotic solution during periods when CVC is not in use) for sterilization and salvage of catheter
  - May decrease relapse of BSI by up to 50%
  - Duration of antibiotic-lock therapy is typically 2 weeks; often used in conjunction with parenteral therapy
  - Lock-therapy is less successful with *Candida* spp and with subcutaneous ports

■ Complications

- Death (20%), septic thrombophlebitis (obtain ultrasound with Doppler, venogram, or CT of affected area), osteomyelitis, endocarditis, suppurative thrombophlebitis, metastatic abscesses

Toxic Shock Syndrome

Toxin mediated, multiorgan-system disease presenting as an acute febrile illness characterized by erythematous eruption and desquamation

■ Epidemiology

- First described in 1978 in seven children with *S. aureus* infection
- A similar toxic shock-like syndrome has been well described in relation to group A streptococcal infection
- Staphylococcal toxic shock syndrome (TSS) epidemic in 1980–1981 statistically linked to use of hyperabsorbency tampons
- 60% of cases occur in young women (ages 15–25); 40% occur in males and nonmenstruating females

■ Risk Factors

- Staphylococcal TSS: Young menstruating female, hyperabsorbency tampon use, vaginal colonization with toxin-producing

S. aureus, focal or surgical wound infection secondary to *S. aureus*, young patients (lack of toxin-neutralizing antibodies)
- Streptococcal TSS: Focal, invasive group A streptococcus, injuries resulting in hematomas, recent surgical procedures, **preceding varicella** or influenza viral infection, all demographic groups effected, most not immunocompromised, slightly increased incidence in alcoholics and diabetics, possible increased prevalence in those using nonsteroidal anti-inflammatory drugs (**NSAIDs**)

■ Etiology
- Common: *S. aureus*, group A *Streptococcus*
- Rare: Groups C, B, D, and G streptococci

■ Pathogenesis
- Exotoxin production; usually toxic shock syndrome toxin-1 (TSST-1; *S. aureus*) or pyrogenic exotoxin A (group A *Streptococcus*, usually M strain types 1 and 3)
- **Toxin acts as superantigen** by stimulating T cells nonspecifically without normal antigenic recognition. Up to one in five T cells activated, whereas only one in 10,000 stimulated during normal antigen presentation
- Cytokine release causes capillary leak with subsequent hypotension

■ History/Physical Exam
- *S. aureus* TSS (Table 15-3)
- Acute febrile illness (over 102°F [38.8°C]) with rash (macular erythroderma followed by late desquamation) and hypotension, and three or more of the following minor criteria:
  - Mucous membrane inflammation (conjunctival, pharyngeal)
  - Abnormalities of the function of the liver, kidneys, central nervous system (coma, obtundation), and gastrointestinal system
  - Muscle abnormalities (myalgias, elevated creatinine phosphokinase levels)
  - Thrombocytopenia

Group A Streptococcus TSS
- Hypotension and shock plus two or more of the following:
  - Renal impairment, DIC, hepatic abnormalities, adult respiratory distress syndrome, scarlet fever rash, soft tissue necrosis
- Isolation of group A *Streptococcus* from a sterile (definitive) or nonsterile (probable) body site

■ **TABLE 15-3   Key Distinguishing Features of Staphylococcal and Streptococcal Toxic Shock Syndromes**

	Staphylococcus aureus	*Streptococcus pyogenes*
Toxin	TSST-1, enterotoxins	SPE A, B
Sex	75% female	Equal distribution
Age	One-third between 15 and 19 years of age	Higher under 4 and over 65 years of age
Key epidemiologic association	Menstruation and tampon use	Varicella infection
Key features		
Prodrome	Vomiting, diarrhea	Flu-like illness
Incidence of prodrome	Common	Less common (20%)
Pain/hyperesthesia	Uncommon	Common
Shock	Predictable	Unpredictable
Focal infection	Less common	Common (75%)
Focal infection, if present	Abscess	Erysipelas or cellulitis, occasionally necrotizing fasciitis
Positive blood culture	Less than 5%	25% to 35%
Multiorgan failure	Correlates with degree of hypotension	Unpredictable
Mortality	3% to 5%	10% to 30% (over 50% if necrotizing fasciitis)

Abbreviations: TSST-1, toxic shock syndrome toxin-1; SPE, streptococcal pyrogenic exotoxin

■ **Additional Studies**

- Blood, mucosal, wound, and vaginal/endocervical cultures: **Assay for toxin production** if *S. aureus* or group A streptococcus isolated (TSST-1-producing *S. aureus* isolated from endocervical cultures in 98% of cases of menstruation-associated TSS but in only 8% to 10% of unaffected women)
- Serum analysis for antibody to exotoxin
- Complete blood count (elevated WBC with increased mature and immature neutrophils; thrombocytopenia)
- Basic metabolic panel (elevated BUN and creatinine secondary to renal dysfunction, also decreased bicarbonate, indicating metabolic acidosis)
- Serum creatinine kinase (increased levels may suggest necrotizing fasciitis or myositis)

- **Plasma lactate:** 3- to 5-fold elevation in severe sepsis (relates to degree of tissue hypoxia; useful for diagnosis and monitoring of therapeutic response)
- **Liver function tests** (elevated serum transaminases and conjugated bilirubin)

■ Differential Diagnosis

- Septic shock, staphylococcal exfoliative syndromes, scarlet fever, Rocky Mountain spotted fever, viral hemorrhagic shock, Stevens-Johnson syndrome, meningococcemia, leptospirosis, and measles

■ Management

- Empiric therapy as for sepsis. Once diagnosis suspected or confirmed, treat with **clindamycin plus oxacillin** (*S. aureus*) **or penicillin** (group A *Streptococcus*)
- Typical course of treatment with beta-lactam antibiotic is **10–14 days** unless focus of infection warrants longer duration of therapy. Clindamycin can be stopped once signs of toxin production abate
- Surgical debridement of abscess or necrotizing fasciitis. Remove tampon if present
- For streptococcal TSS, consider adding intravenous immune globulin (IVIG). Well-controlled clinical trials to date have insufficient power to demonstrate clear benefit

■ Complications (see Table 15-3 for mortality)

- Staphylococcal TSS
  - Recurrence of both menstrual and nonmenstrual TSS described (women should not use tampons for five menstrual cycles and should complete a full course of antibiotics)
  - Persistent neuropsychological alteration (memory loss, lack of concentration, abnormal electroencephalogram [EEG])
  - Mild, persistent renal failure
- Streptococcal TSS
  - **Bacteremia common** (where it is rare in *S. aureus* TSS)
  - Aggressive soft tissue infection
  - Shock, ARDS, renal failure

16

Human Immunodeficiency Virus

Heidi M. Crane, MD, MPH and
Mari M. Kitahata, MD, MPH

- HIV infection is caused by human immunodeficiency viruses (HIV-1 and HIV-2) from the family of human retroviruses and the subfamily of lentiviruses
- **Acquired immunodeficiency syndrome** (AIDS) is defined by the Centers for Disease Control (CDC) to include any HIV-infected person with any of 26 clinical conditions (Table 16-1)
- AIDS also includes any HIV-infected person with a CD4+ T-lymphocyte cell count (CD4+ count) **below 200 cells/mm^3**

■ Epidemiology

- Over 50 million people worldwide have been infected with HIV
- Sub-Saharan Africa is the most severely affected area
  - In Botswana and Zimbabwe, HIV prevalence rates are over 30%
- Over 900,000 persons are living with HIV in the US
  - As many as ¼ are unaware of their infection
  - The epidemic is growing fastest among minority populations
  - Leading killer of African-American males aged 25–44
  - Compared to whites, HIV prevalence is nearly seven times higher among African-Americans and three times higher among Hispanics

■ HIV Transmission and Risk Factors

- Transmission via infected fluids such as blood (sharing of needles by intravenous drug users), homosexual and heterosexual contact, and by infected mothers to infants either intrapartum, perinatally, or via breast milk
- Genital ulcers and other sexually transmitted diseases increase transmission rates
- Risk of **mother-to-child transmission** increases with high viral load, low CD4+ count, preterm delivery, chorioamnionitis, breastfeeding, and prolonged rupture of membranes
- Vertical transmission rate if mother is not on therapy is ~25%

■ TABLE 16-1   HIV/AIDS Classification System

CD4+ Count (Cells/mm³ of Blood)	Category A	Category B	Category C
	Asymptomatic	Symptomatic[a]	Symptomatic[b]
≥500	A1	B1	C1
200–499	A2	B2	C2
<200	A3	B3	C3

All patients in A3, B3, and C1 to C3 (non-shaded areas) have AIDS (due to an AIDS-defining illness or a CD4+ count below 200/mm³)

[a] Category B symptoms: Any HIV-related symptom NOT on category C list
[b] Category C symptoms: Opportunistic infections, certain malignancies, wasting

- Vertical transmission rate if mother is on highly active anti-retroviral therapy (HAART) is less than 5%
- Risk of acquiring HIV from a transfusion in the US is one in 676,000

■ Pathogenesis

- HIV envelope glycoproteins bind with CD4+ cell
- HIV nucleoprotein complex enters cytoplasm
- Transcription of RNA viral genome by viral reverse transcriptase
- Resulting double-stranded viral DNA enters nucleus and integrates with host chromosome catalyzed by integrase
- Viral replication occurs and virions are released by budding. This is lytic to infected CD4+ cells
- Rapid production and destruction of CD4+ cells
- The fall in CD4+ count (in cells/mm³) is a measure of the extent of immune dysfunction

■ Postexposure Prophylaxis (PEP)

- Factors that increase the **risk of occupational exposure** include: Hollow needle, visible blood, deep injury, needle used in artery or vein
- For high-risk occupational exposures, use two- or three-drug regimens for 4 weeks (often Combivir [AZT/3TC] in addition to a protease inhibitor)
- Drug regimen based on source of patient's prior antiretroviral treatment and resistance if known
- PEP should be started immediately (no benefit after 72 hours)
- **Laboratory tests for patients starting PEP:**
  - At baseline: HIV enzyme-linked immunosorbent assay (ELISA)/Western blot, complete blood count (CBC),

■ **BOX 16-1   Clinical Features of Primary HIV Infection**

Common
Fever (97%)

Lymphadenopathy (77%)

Pharyngitis (73%)

Maculopapular rash (70%)

Arthralgias/myalgias (58%)

Less Common
Mucocutaneous ulceration (35%)

Diarrhea (33%)

Headache (30%)

Oral candidiasis (10%)

comprehensive metabolic panel (CMP; includes electrolytes, BUN/creatinine, liver function tests), hepatitis B and C serologies
- At 2 weeks: CBC, CMP for potential drug toxicity
- Repeat HIV ELISA/Western blot (and hepatitis serologies as appropriate) at 6, 12, and 24 weeks
• Limited data on use of PEP in nonoccupational settings

■ **Natural History**

• Stages of HIV infection: Transmission, acute retroviral syndrome, asymptomatic infection, then symptomatic AIDS
• Disease progression varies greatly among individuals. Estimated time from transmission to death without antiretroviral therapy approximately 10–11 years
• Acute primary HIV is often symptomatic. Can mimic mononucleosis. See Box 16-1 for symptoms. Usually not diagnosed. Important to make diagnosis for early intervention and education for patients that they are at risk of spreading disease
• HIV RNA (viral load) increases during acute infection and then declines to a new "set point" for period of years and then gradually increases. CD4+ counts gradually decrease

■ **Initial Evaluation for HIV-Infected Patient**

• Discuss HIV knowledge base, risk factors and transmission prevention strategies, HIV history (CD4+ counts, HIV RNA level, opportunistic infections, prior antiretroviral therapy)
• Review all medications
• Perform thorough physical exam, including a cervical Papanicolaou (Pap) smear for women

Indication	Prophylaxis	Indication to Stop Primary Prophylaxis
TABLE 16-2 Opportunistic Infection Prophylaxis		
Pneumocystis jiroveci CD4+ count < 200 or history of thrush	First choice: TMP/SMX 1 double strength or single strength PO daily	CD4+ count > 200 for 3 months
	Second choice: If allergic, dapsone 100 mg PO daily	
	Third choice: Aerosolized pentamidine 300 mg monthly	
Toxoplasma gondii CD4+ count < 100 and positive *Toxoplasma* IgG	First choice: TMP/SMX 1 double strength or single strength PO daily	CD4+ count > 200 for 3 months
Mycobacterium tuberculosis **(latent disease)** PPD positive (≥5 mm induration) without active TB	Many regimens, but first choice: Isoniazid 300 mg + pyridoxine 50 mg PO daily for 9 months	Duration varies, often 9-month course
Mycobacterium avium complex **(MAC)** CD4+ count < 50	Azithromycin 1200 mg PO weekly or clarithromycin 500 mg PO twice daily	CD4+ count > 100 for 3 months

Abbreviations: TMP/SMX, trimethoprim-sulfamethoxazole

- Check labs: HIV enzyme immunosorbent assay (EIA or ELISA) and Western blot (if HIV infection not satisfactorily documented); CD4+ count; HIV RNA level; CBC; CMP; lipid panel; *Toxoplasma gondii* IgG; syphilis test (RPR); hepatitis A, B, and C serologies; sexually transmissible disease (STD) screen
- Place TB test (PPD), give routine immunizations as needed (pneumococcus, hepatitis A and B, and influenza)

■ **Opportunistic Infection (OI) Prophylaxis** (Table 16-2)

■ **Initiating Antiretroviral Therapy** (see also Chapter 5)

- Initiation of antiretroviral medications should be performed in consultation with an expert in HIV care, in collaboration with the patient, considering:
  - Willingness/readiness of patient
  - Degree of existing immunodeficiency (CD4+ count)
  - Risk for disease progression (CD4+ count and HIV RNA level)
  - Potential risks and benefits
  - Compliance with medication regimens

- **Treatment** should usually be offered to:
  - Symptomatic HIV-infected patients
  - Patients who have a CD4+ count of 350 or less
  - Patients who have an HIV RNA level over 55,000 copies/mL
- Treatment **goals** should be:
  - Maximal and durable suppression of HIV RNA level
  - Restoration of immune function/CD4+ count
  - Improvement in quality of life
  - Reduction of HIV-related morbidity and mortality

■ HIV Antibody Testing and Disease Monitoring

- Pre- and post-test risk reduction counseling with HIV testing

ELISA

- Sensitive, specific, rare false positives occur, not sufficient without Western Blot confirmation
- May be negative first few weeks to months after infection

HIV Western Blot

- Used as a confirmatory test if ELISA positive
- More specific than ELISA

Quantitative HIV RNA Level (Viral Load)

- Diagnose acute HIV before antibody tests become positive (requires follow-up confirmation)
- Predict rate of progression (higher HIV RNA level set point is associated with faster rates of disease progression)
- Therapeutic monitoring (change of >0.5 log copies/mL exceeds assay/diurnal variation and is not random variability)

CD4+ Cell Count (Table 16-3)

- Normal > 750 cells/mm^3
- Determine disease stage, monitor effect on immune system, make therapeutic decisions, and predict prognosis
  - CD4+ count < 350: Immune function impairment
  - CD4+ count < 200: Imminent risk of OIs

■ TABLE 16-3 HIV Interventions Based on CD4+ Cell Count	
CD4+ Cell Count, Cells/mm³	**Intervention**
<350	Consider initiating HAART
<200	PCP prophylaxis
<100	Toxoplasmosis prophylaxis
<50	MAC prophylaxis

■ **BOX 16-2   CD4+ Counts of Common Infections**

CD4+ Count > 200 Cells/mm³
Herpes zoster

TB

Oral hairy leukoplakia

Recurrent bacterial pneumonia

Oral candidiasis

CD4+ Count < 200 Cells/mm³
Pneumocystis jiroveci pneumonia (PCP)

Candida esophagitis

Cytomegalovirus (CMV) retinitis, colitis*

T. gondii encephalitis*

MAC*

Cryptococcal meningitis*

* Usually occur in patients with CD4+ counts < 100 cells/mm³

- A "train on a track" analogy can describe the independent contributions of CD4+ counts and HIV RNA level. If a person is imagined as being on a train traveling toward a clinical event such as acquiring an OI or dying from AIDS, the CD4+ count describes the distance from the destination, and the viral load describes the speed with which the train is traveling to the destination

■ **Common Complications** (Box 16-2)

Pulmonary Complications
- *Pneumocystis carinii* pneumonia (PCP) recently renamed *P. jiroveci*
  - Fever, nonproductive cough, progressive dyspnea
  - Often marked decrease in arterial partial pressure of oxygen (PaO_2) and increase in alveolar-arterial (A-a) gradient
  - **Hypoxemia** often worse than chest x-ray (CXR) appearance would suggest
  - **Diffuse or perihilar infiltrates** on CXR, 10% to 20% with normal CXR, usually "ground glass" appearance on CT
  - Trimethoprim 15 mg/kg/day + sulfamethoxazole 75 mg/kg/day for 21 days
  - If hypoxemic (PaO_2 < 70 mmHg or A-a gradient > 35 mmHg), give patients prednisone 40 mg PO twice daily for 5 days, then taper

- **TB** (may be PPD anergic; see also Chapter 9)
  - Can occur at any HIV disease stage
  - Unusual presentations in patients with advanced HIV: Lower lobe involvement, adenopathy, extrapulmonary disease

Gastrointestinal Complications
- **Esophagitis**
  - Most often candidal esophagitis, especially in patients with oral thrush
    - Treat empirically with fluconazole 200 mg (up to 800 mg) PO daily for 2–3 weeks
    - If no response, perform esophagogastroduodenoscopy (EGD)
  - If ulcers: CMV (45%) > aphthous ulcers (40%) > herpes simplex virus (HSV; 5%)
- **Drug-related diarrhea**
  - Often associated with nelfinavir, lopinavir/ritonavir (protease inhibitors)
  - Treatment: Loperamide; if no response, consider stopping offending drug
- **Chronic diarrhea** (more than 30 days)
  - CMV (15% to 40% of chronic diarrhea in patients with AIDS)
    - CD4+ count below 50
    - Colitis or enteritis, requires biopsy for diagnosis
  - *Cryptosporidia* (15% to 30% of chronic diarrhea)
    - Diagnosis by oocysts in stool
    - Often resolves with HAART
  - *Mycobacterium avium complex* (CD4+ count below 50)
    - Can cause diarrhea, abdominal pain, adenopathy, hepatosplenomegaly, wasting, and fever
    - Diagnosis by positive blood cultures (versus biopsy)
    - Clarithromycin 500 mg PO twice daily + ethambutol 15 mg/kg/day
  - Other causes of chronic diarrhea in patients with AIDS include *Cyclospora, Entamoeba histolytica, Giardia lamblia, Microsporidia*

Dermatology/Oral
- **Oral ulcers:** Most often aphthous ulcers or HSV
- **Oral hairy leukoplakia**
  - Associated with Epstein-Barr virus
  - White patches on side of tongue, specific marker for HIV
  - Does not scrape off (unlike thrush), no treatment needed
- **Oral candidiasis** (also called thrush)
  - Three types: Erythematous, pseudomembranous, angular cheilitis

- Can scrape off, check KOH stain for diagnosis
- Indicator of need for PCP prophylaxis
- Fluconazole 200 mg (up to 800 mg) PO daily until lesions resolve
- **Kaposi's sarcoma**
  - Cause by human herpesvirus type 8 (HHV-8)
  - Firm, purple to brownish-black lesions
  - Visceral involvement common
  - Diagnosis by appearance, biopsy if atypical
  - Often improves with HAART, may require chemotherapy
- **Seborrheic dermatitis**
  - Especially common on scalp, central face, and behind ears
  - Diagnosis based on typical appearance
  - Topical steroids + topical antifungal (ketoconazole)

Metabolic
- **Lipodystrophy**
  - Typically develops in patients on antiretroviral therapy
  - Thin face (may have sunken cheeks, temporal wasting) and thin extremities (peripheral lipoatrophy), central adiposity (lipohypertrophy), dyslipidemia, insulin resistance
  - Consider changing antiretroviral medications

Neurologic
- **Peripheral neuropathy**
  - Often associated with antiretrovirals: Stavudine (d4T), didanosine (ddI), zalcitabine (ddC)
  - May improve with discontinuation of offending drug
- **AIDS dementia complex**
  - Poor concentration, diminished memory, slowing of thought processes and motor dysfunction
  - May improve with HAART
- **Toxoplasmosis** (CD4+ count below 100)
  - Subacute symptoms with fever, headache, behavior change
  - MRI with ring enhancing lesions and edema
  - Positive *T. gondii* IgG > 90%
  - Cerebrospinal fluid (CSF) *T. gondii* PCR: 50% sensitive, > 96% specific
  - Clinical and MRI response to pyrimethamine and sulfadiazine treatment within 2 weeks
- **Cytomegalovirus encephalitis** (CD4+ count below 50)
  - Rapidly progressive delirium, cranial nerve defects, ataxia, headache, fever
  - MRI with periventricular lesions and enhancement
  - Diagnosis: CMV PCR in cerebrospinal fluid
  - Treatment: Ganciclovir/foscarnet and HAART
- **Cytomegalovirus retinitis** (CD4+ count below 50)

- Blurring, blind spots, flashing lights, central vision loss
- Diagnosis: Typical appearance on funduscopic exam
- Treatment: HAART, intraocular ganciclovir, valganciclovir

Hematologic Complications
- **Anemia**
  - Drug-induced: Zidovudine (AZT) most common (macrocytic)
  - Marrow infiltration: MAC, lymphoma, TB, CMV
  - Other: HIV, iron/nutritional deficiency, parvovirus B19
- **Non-Hodgkin's lymphoma**
  - More than 200 times as common in patients with HIV
  - May present as fever of unknown origin, diagnosis by biopsy
  - Most are high-grade diffuse large cell or Burkitt's-like lymphomas
  - Treatment: Chemotherapy and HAART

17 Infections in Special Hosts

Mari Mizuta, MD

Fever and Neutropenia

- Oral temperature 38.3°C (101°F) or above with absolute neutrophil count (ANC) of less than 500 cells/mm³, or less than 1000 cells/mm³ and decreasing (decrease to below 500 cells/mm³ anticipated)
- ANC equals the total white blood cell (WBC) count multiplied by the percentage of neutrophils and bands

■ Epidemiology
- Half of febrile neutropenic patients have an established or occult infection

■ Risk Factors
- Profound/prolonged neutropenia
- Mucositis
- Damage to the skin by invasive procedure (e.g., vascular access device placement, phlebotomy)
- Impaired cellular immunity due to malignancy or chemotherapy

■ Etiology
- Common bacteria (see Box 17-1)
- Gram-positive bacteria account for up to 70% of documented infections (catheter-related bacteremia, cellulitis, etc.)
- Typhlitis, cecitis, *Clostridium difficile* colitis
- Candidemia, candida esophagitis, hematogenously disseminated candidiasis (liver, kidney, brain)
- *Aspergillus*, less commonly other moulds: Pneumonia, sinusitis, brain abscess
- *Pneumocystis jiroveci* (formerly *P. carinii*) pneumonitis
- Herpes simplex virus (HSV): Stomatitis, esophagitis; rarely pneumonitis, hepatitis, or encephalitis
- Varicella-zoster virus (VZV): Shingles, rarely visceral dissemination

■ **BOX 17-1   Common Bacterial Causes of Febrile Neutropenia**

Gram-Positive Bacteria
Staphylococcus spp

Streptococcus spp

Enterococcus spp

Corynebacterium spp

Gram-Negative Bacteria
Escherichia coli

Klebsiella spp

Pseudomonas aeruginosa

■ **Pathogenesis**

- Invasion of bacteria from alimentary tract with chemotherapy-induced mucosal damage
- Bacterial entrance from damaged skin
- Respiratory inhalation (*Aspergillus* spp)
- Reactivation of pathogens (HSV, VZV, *P. jiroveci*)

■ **History/Physical Exam**

- Signs and/or symptoms of inflammation may be minimal or absent
  - Cellulitis with only minimal induration, erythema, and pustulation
  - Pulmonary infection without infiltrates
  - Meningitis without cerebrospinal fluid (CSF) pleocytosis
  - Urinary tract infection (UTI) without pyuria
- Search for subtle symptoms and signs
  - Pay special attention to skin (including catheter site), fundus, periodontium, pharynx, lung, perineum, anus
  - Cough, pleuritic chest pain, hemoptysis suggest invasive pulmonary aspergillosis
  - Facial swelling, ophthalmoplegia suggest fungal sinusitis

■ **Additional Studies**

- Complete blood count (CBC) with differential
- Blood culture (see also Chapter 15)
- Urinalysis, urine culture
- Chest x-ray (CXR)
- Serum electrolytes, BUN, creatinine, hepatic transaminases
- Chest CT: Halo sign is highly specific for invasive *Aspergillus*
- Sputum culture, bronchoscopy with lavage, ±biopsy
- Sinus CT, nasal endoscopy ± biopsy

- HSV- and VZV-direct fluorescent antibody (DFA) of suspicious mucocutaneous lesions
- Abdomen and pelvis CT
- C. *difficile* toxins A and B with diarrhea
- Lumbar puncture if meningitis is suspected

■ Differential Diagnosis

- Drug fever, tumor fever, transfusion reaction, thromboembolic disease, radiation reaction, pulmonary hemorrhage

■ Management

- Promptly start empirical antibiotic therapy following guidelines for use of antimicrobial agents in neutropenic patients with cancer prepared by the Infectious Diseases Society of America (described below)
- In low-risk patients (no appearance of illness, no alteration of mental status, no focus of infection, normal CXR, duration of neutropenia less than 7 days, ANC 100/mm^3 or higher, no local CVC-site infection, resolution of neutropenia expected to occur within 10 days) consideration can be made to closely follow as outpatients
- High-risk patients: Mucositis, hemodynamic instability, ANC below 100/mm^3 require admission

Initial Empirical Antimicrobial Regimens

- Low-risk patients should receive oral ciprofloxacin plus amoxicillin-clavulanate or IV antibiotics as described below
- High-risk patients should receive IV antibiotics as described below
- Monotherapy: Cefepime, ceftazidime, or carbapenem (imipenem-cilastatin or meropenem)
- Dual therapy: Cefepime, ceftazidime, carbapenem, or antipseudomonal aminopenicillins (ticarcillin-clavulanate or piperacillin-tazobactam) plus aminoglycoside (gentamicin, tobramycin, amikacin) in complicated cases or in institutions with resistance problems
- **Vancomycin is not routinely added** (risk of vancomycin-resistant *Enterococcus* [VRE] emergence). Use in cases of:
  - Suspected serious catheter-related infection
  - Known colonization with methicillin-resistant *Staphylococcus aureus* (MRSA)
  - Known penicillin and cephalosporin-resistant pneumococci
  - Cellulitis or mucositis
  - Positive blood culture for gram-positive organisms
  - Hypotension
  - Frequent serious infections with gram-positive organisms in the institution

Afebrile in 3–5 Days

- If infectious etiology is identified, antibiotics should be adjusted appropriately based on site of infection and results of antibiotic susceptibility testing (when organism isolated). Antipseudomonal coverage should be maintained at least until resolution of neutropenia
- If no identified infection:
  - Initially at low risk, may change to oral ciprofloxacin plus amoxicillin-clavulanate, after afebrile for 48 hours
  - Initially at high risk, continue the same antibiotics
- Duration of therapy:
  - If infectious etiology is identified, duration depends on infection but treat at least for 7 days until ANC over $500/mm^3$
  - If no identified infection:
    - ANC over $500/mm^3$, treat until afebrile and ANC has been over $500/mm^3$ for more than 48 hours
    - ANC less than $500/mm^3$ by day 7: If initially low risk, stop therapy when afebrile for 5–7 days or when ANC is above $500/mm^3$. If initially high risk, continue therapy until resolution of neutropenia

Persistent Fever Throughout the First 3–5 Days

- Reassessment: Review all previous culture results, meticulous physical exam, CXR, additional cultures of blood and any other potential sites of infection
- Consider CT of head, sinuses, chest, or abdomen; or ultrasound of abdomen (concern for sinusitis, pneumonitis, cecitis)
- If not clinically worsening, continue same antibiotics. Stop vancomycin if there is no evidence for gram-positive infections
- If clinically worsening, change antibiotics
- Consider adding an antifungal drug (amphotericin B, caspofungin, or voriconazole) after day 5
- Duration of therapy:
  - If infection is identified, duration depends on the infection
  - If no identified infection:
    - ANC over $500/mm^3$: Stop therapy after ANC has been above $500/mm^3$ for 4–5 days
    - ANC below $500/mm^3$: Reassess and continue therapy for 2 weeks, then reassess and consider stopping therapy if no infection is found

Specific Nonbacterial Therapy

- *Candida* spp: Fluconazole if sensitive strain, and amphotericin B, voriconazole, or caspofungin for resistant strains (see also Chapter 4)
- Aspergillus: Amphotericin B or voriconazole

- HSV, VZV: Acyclovir
- *P. jiroveci:* Trimethoprim-sulfamethoxazole (TMP/SMX)

Adjunctive Measures
- Granulocyte colony-stimulating factor (GCSF) shortens duration of neutropenia, but no change in other outcomes. Consider if clinical worsening is predicted
- Granulocyte transfusions may be helpful in documented bacterial or fungal infections not controlled by antibiotics and GCSF
- **Antimicrobial prophylaxis is not routinely recommended because of emerging resistance, except for the use of TMP/SMX for *P. jiroveci***

Infections in Solid Organ Transplants

■ Epidemiology

- Frequency of infection based on type of transplanted organ and extent of immunosuppression required to prevent organ rejection
  - Risk of infection: Heart-lung transplant (lung infection) > lung (lung) > liver (abdomen and biliary system) > heart (lung) > kidney (UTI)

■ Risk Factors

- Net exposure to pathogen: Prior colonization, pathogens from donor, and nosocomial exposure
- Net state of immunosuppression: Immunosuppressive agents, underlying immune deficiency, neutropenia, disruption of mucocutaneous barriers, and infection with immunomodulating viruses (cytomegalovirus [CMV], Epstein-Barr virus [EBV], hepatitis B virus [HBV], hepatitis C virus [HCV], HIV)

■ Etiology

Types of Infections After Transplantation (see Table 17-1)
- Phase 1: First month after transplantation
  - More than 90% are conventional nosocomial infections such as bacterial and fungal infections of surgical wound, lungs, urinary tract, and vascular access devices
  - Recurrence of infection present in donor or recipient
- Phase 2: 1–6 months after transplantation
  - Unconventional or opportunistic infections
- Phase 3: More than 6 months after transplantation
  - 80% of patients are on minimal immunosuppression: At risk for conventional community-acquired infections
  - 10% have chronic or progression with viruses
  - 10% have recurrent or chronic rejection requiring more immunosuppression (at risk for infections seen in phase 2)

■ **TABLE 17-1   Common Infections After Organ Transplantation**

	Less than 1 Month	1–6 Months	More than 6 Months
Bacterial	Nosocomial	*Nocardia*	
	Donor origin	*Listeria*	
		Mycobacteria tuberculosis	
Viral	HSV	CMV, EBV, VZV	CMV
	HBV	HBV, HCV	PTLD
	HCV	Respiratory viruses	Papillomavirus
Fungal	*Candida*	Pneumocystis	Endemic mycoses
		Aspergillus	(*Histoplasma,*
		Cryptococcus neoformans	*Coccidioides,*
Parasitic		*Strongyloides*	*Blastomyces*)
		Toxoplasma	
		Leishmania	
		Trypanosoma	

Abbreviations: CMV, cytomegalovirus; EBV, Epstein-Barr virus; HBV, hepatitis B virus; HCV, hepatitis C virus; HSV, herpes simplex virus; PTLD, posttransplantation lymphoproliferative disorder; VZV, varicella-zoster virus

Cytomegalovirus
- Effects:
  - Cytopenia, hepatitis, pneumonitis, colitis, encephalitis
  - Allograft infection by CMV
  - Allograft injury and rejection
  - Enhancement of systemic immunosuppression
  - EBV-associated post-transplantation lymphoproliferative disorder (PTLD)

Post-Transplantation Lymphoproliferative Disorder
- **Associated with EBV proliferation**
- Primary EBV infection is a particular risk
- Ranges from B-cell benign polyclonal proliferation to highly malignant monoclonal lymphoma
- Often extranodal (brain, bone marrow, allograft, GI tract, liver)

Common Infections After Liver Transplantation
- Liver abscess, cholangitis
- Reactivation of HBV, HCV

Common Infections After Kidney Transplantation
- UTI
- BK virus infection: Hemorrhagic cystitis, ureteric obstruction, renal failure

Miscellaneous Infections (see also Neutropenia, below)
- *Toxoplasma:* Myocarditis, encephalitis, chorioretinitis
- Parvovirus B19: Anemia
- Human herpesvirus 6 (HHV-6): Cytopenia, meningoencephalitis
- HHV-8: Kaposi's sarcoma
- Adenovirus: Pneumonitis, hepatitis, cystitis, dissemination
- *Strongyloides stercoralis* (reactivation): Hyperinfection syndrome (augmentation of normal helminth life cycle with massive infestation of the GI tract and lungs and potential dissemination to other organs). May be associated with pneumonia, enterocolitis, and gram-negative sepsis

■ Pathogenesis
- Reactivation of donor- or recipient-origin pathogens
- Nosocomial or community-acquired pathogens
- Proliferation of these pathogens under immunosuppression

■ History/Physical Exam
- Type of transplant
- Underlying medical conditions
- Posttransplant course (including infections, rejections, immunosuppression)
- Search for subtle symptoms and signs

■ Additional Studies
- Complete blood count with differential
- Complete metabolic panel including liver function tests
- Blood cultures
- Urinalysis, urine culture
- CXR
- Brain CT/MRI, sinus CT, chest CT, abdomen CT/ultrasound as indicated
- CMV antigenemia or PCR (serology has little role), tissue biopsy (for histology, PCR, and shell vial culture)
- EBV PCR
- Respiratory virus (influenza, parainfluenza, RSV, adenovirus): Enzyme immunoassay or fluorescent antibody test of nasopharyngeal swab
- Bronchoscopy ± alveolar lavage ± biopsy, transthoracic or thoracoscopic biopsy for culture, histology

- CSF cell counts, glucose, protein, staining/culture (bacterial, fungal, acid-fast bacilli), cryptococcal antigen, viral PCRs, brain biopsy
- BK virus urine cytology and PCR
- Adenovirus culture or antigen detection
- Parvovirus PCR

■ **Differential Diagnosis**

- Pulmonary lesions (Box 17-2) and brain lesions (Box 17-3)
- Common noninfectious differentials: Drug effect, rejection, thromboembolic disease

---

▨ BOX 17-2   Differential Diagnosis of Lung Lesions After Transplant

Bacterial
Community-acquired pneumonia
Legionella
M. tuberculosis
Nocardia
Antinomyces

Fungal
P. jiroveci
Aspergillus
Endemic mycoses
Cryptococcus

Viral
Respiratory viruses*
CMV
HSV
VZV

Noninfectious
Thromboembolism
Hemorrhage
Edema
Leukoaggregation
Drug reaction
Tumor
Rejection (lung)

*Respiratory viruses include adenovirus, influenza viruses A and B, parainfluenza viruses, and respiratory syncytial virus

■ **BOX 17-3   Differential Diagnosis of Brain Lesions After Transplant**

Bacterial
Listeria
Nocardia
Antinomyces
M. tuberculosis
Brain abscess

Fungal
Cryptococcus
Aspergillus
Endemic mycoses

Viral
EBV (PTLD)
HSV
CMV
VZV
JC virus (progressive multifocal leukoencephalopathy)
Parasitic
Toxoplasma gondii

Noninfectious
Toxic drug effect
Hemorrhage
Ischemia
Tumor
Vasculitis

■ Management

Treatment
- CMV: Intravenous ganciclovir until viremia clears
- PTLD: Reduction of immunosuppression and chemotherapy
- Polyoma virus (BK virus, JC virus): reduction of immunosuppression
- RSV: Aerosolized ribavirin, ±RSV immunoglobulin

Prophylaxis
- *P. jiroveci:* TMP/SMX until immunosuppression is reduced; life-long for lung transplant recipients (effective also for toxoplasmosis, nocardiosis, listeriosis, and UTI)
- CMV: Ganciclovir or valgancyclovir for at-risk patients (all except donor negative-recipient negative cases)
- HSV: Acyclovir (unnecessary if on ganciclovir)

■ **Complications**

- Organ failure/rejection (need for retransplant), death

Infections in Bone Marrow Transplants

■ **Epidemiology**

- Phase 1 (0–30 days): Pre-engraftment phase
- Phase 2 (30–100 days): Postengraftment phase
- Phase 3 (>100 days): Late phase
- Engraftment = ANC over $500/mm^3$ after transplant
- Autologous bone marrow recipients are at greatest risk in phase 1

■ **Risk Factors**

Phase 1

- Neutropenia
- Breaks in mucocutaneous barriers due to preparative regimens and frequent vascular access

Phase 2

- **Impaired cell-mediated immunity**
- Graft-versus-host disease (GVHD)
- Immunosuppressive therapy for GVHD

Phase 3

- **Humoral-immunity defect**
- Impaired reticuloendothelial system function
- GVHD
- Immunosuppressive therapy for GVHD

■ **Etiology** (See Box 17-4)

■ **Pathogenesis**

- Reactivation of pathogens
- Nosocomial or community-acquired pathogens
- Proliferation of these pathogens under immunosuppression

■ **History/Physical Exam**

- Type of transplant (allogenic or autologous); increased risk with allogenic transplant
- Underlying medical conditions
- Posttransplant course (including infections, GVHD, immunosuppression)
- Search for subtle symptoms and signs

■ **Additional Studies** (see also Infections in Solid Organ Transplants, above)

- CBC with differential

■ BOX 17-4   Common Infections After Bone Marrow Transplant

0–30 days
HSV
Candida
Aspergillus
Nosocomial bacteria

30–100 days
CMV
Pneumocystis
Aspergillus

>100 days
CMV
VZV
EBV-PTLD
Respiratory viruses
Encapsulated bacteria

- Complete metabolic panel including liver function tests
- Blood cultures
- Urinalysis, urine culture
- CXR
- Galactomannon antigen ELISA (approved blood test for invasive *Aspergillus*): sensitivity 65% to 93%, specificity 95% (false positive result may occur in patients receiving piperacillin-tazobactam)

■ Differential Diagnosis
- Drug fever
- Thromboembolic disease
- Interstitial pneumonitis
- Veno-occlusive disease (VOD) of liver seen up to day 20
- Diffuse alveolar hemorrhage
- Bronchiolitis obliterans
- GVHD (skin, GI tract)

■ Management
Treatment
- CMV: During phase 2, select either (1) prophylaxis with ganciclovir or valganciclovir or (2) routine weekly screening for

antigenemia or virus excretion (DNA-PCR). If detectable pre-emptively treat with ganciclovir
- Ganciclovir plus intravenous immunoglobulin (IVIG) for CMV pneumonitis
- Granulocyte-macrophage colony-stimulating factor
- Granulocyte transfusion in severe infections

Prophylaxis
- CMV: Leukocyte-reduced blood products if both donor and recipient were CMV IgG-negative
- HSV: Acyclovir until engraftment or mucositis resolves in HSV IgG-positive patients
- Candida: Fluconazole until day 75
- *Pneumocystis:* TMP/SMX or dapsone from engraftment until 6 months or longer if has chronic GVHD

■ Complications
- Multiorgan failure, death

Postsplenectomy Sepsis

■ Epidemiology
- Infection rate: 3.2%
- More common in children

■ Risk Factors
- **50% of sepsis cases occur within 2 years of splenectomy, but the risk is lifelong**
- A third of cases occur more than 5 years after splenectomy
- Infection risk varies by underlying disease: Thalassemia major > sickle cell anemia > Hodgkin's disease > spherocytosis > trauma > idiopathic thrombocytopenic purpura
- Current immunosuppressive therapy or radiation therapy
- Special exposures to etiologic organisms (e.g., *Babesia, Plasmodium, Capnocytophaga*)

■ Etiology
- **Encapsulated bacteria** (by far the most important): *Streptococcus pneumoniae* (66%), *Haemophilus influenzae,* and *Neisseria meningitidis*
- Gram-negative rods: *E. coli, Pseudomonas aeruginosa, Salmonella*
- Others: *Babesia, Plasmodium, Capnocytophaga, Bartonella*

■ Pathogenesis
- Lack of splenic opsonization and phagocytic function
- Reduced immune regulation

■ History/Physical Exam

- Fever, chills, rigors
- Hypotension
- Vomiting, diarrhea
- Seizure, coma, neck stiffness (suggests meningitis)
- Purpura (suggests disseminated intravascular coagulation)
- Rapid deterioration
- Travel history, exposure to animals

■ Additional Studies

- Blood cultures
- Blood smear (Gram stain is often positive due to high degree of bacteremia, Giemsa stain for *Plasmodium* and *Babesia*)
- CSF cell count, glucose, protein, Gram stain, and culture if meningitis is suspected
- Gram stain and culture of rash
- Complete blood count (leukocytosis, thrombocytopenia)
- Serum electrolytes, BUN, creatinine, prothrombin time (PT), partial thromboplastin time (PTT), D-dimers or fibrinogen and fibrin split products
- CXR

■ Management

- **Prompt antibiotic administration (do not wait for diagnostic studies), usually ceftriaxone**
  - Add vancomycin in severely ill patients
- Some advise immediate self-treatment with amoxicillin at symptom onset, with immediate medical follow-up
- Prophylaxis with amoxicillin (erythromycin in case of penicillin allergy) is not commonly given for adults
- Immunizations, especially against *S. pneumoniae* should be given prior to splenectomy

■ Complications

- DIC, multiorgan failure
- Mortality: 60%

Infections During Pregnancy — Bacteriuria

See Table 17-2 for other infections during pregnancy

■ Epidemiology

- Bacteriuria is the most common infection during pregnancy
- Found in 4% to 7% of pregnant women

■ TABLE 17-2   Important Infections During Pregnancy

Maternal Infections	Complications	Remarks
Toxoplasma	Congenital toxoplasmosis	Spiramycin to prevent fetal transmission
		If already transmitted to fetus, pyrimethamine + sulfadiazine
Syphilis	Congenital syphilis	Penicillin
		If allergic, desensitize
Rubella	Congenital rubella syndrome	Rare in US because of vaccination
CMV	Congenital CMV	Most common congenital viral infection
HSV (genital)	Neonatal skin infection	Much more severe with primary infection
	CNS infection	
	Dissemination	Highest risk at or near labor
Chlamydia, Gonorrhea, Trichomonas	Abortion, PROM, LBW infant Prematurity	Neonatal conjunctivitis (gonorrhea and chlamydia) *Chlamydia pneumoniae*
Listeria bacteremia	Premature labor	Predisposition: Impaired cell-mediated immunity during pregnancy
	22% stillbirth	
	Neonatal death	Meningitis is rare
Group B streptococcus	Amnionitis	Leading infectious cause of neonatal mortality and morbidity
	PROM	
	Neonatal bacteremia, pneumonia, meningitis	Vaginal and rectal screening at 35–37 weeks
		Intrapartum chemoprophylaxis with penicillin (clindamycin, erythromycin, or vancomycin if allergic)
Parvovirus B19	Hydrops fetalis	

Abbreviations: CMV, cytomegalovirus; CNS, central nervous system; HSV, herpes simplex virus; LBW, low birth weight; PROM, premature rupture of membranes

■ Risk Factors

- Older age, parity, lower socioeconomic status, frequent sexual activity, diabetes, sickle cell trait, history of UTI

■ Etiology

- Same microbiologic picture as in nonpregnant cases (*E. coli* is by far the most common)

■ Pathogenesis

- Decreased ureteral peristalsis
- Decreased bladder tone
- Dilatation of ureter and renal pelvis
- Ascending route of infection

■ History/Physical Exam

- Usually asymptomatic (detected during screening)
- Fever, chills
- Dysuria, frequency
- Abdominal pain, back pain
- History of UTI
- Frequent sexual activity

■ Additional Studies

- Urinalysis
- Urine culture
- Blood cultures if pyelonephritis is suspected

■ Management

- **Antimicrobials even if asymptomatic**
- 7-day course of treatment based on urine culture sensitivity results (amoxicillin is given most commonly)
- Longer course is required for pyelonephritis
- Repeat urine culture after treatment to confirm sterility

■ Complications

- If untreated, 20% to 40% of asymptomatic bacteriuria will progress to pyelonephritis later in the pregnancy
- Chorioamnionitis, septicemia, preeclampsia
- Premature delivery (50% are due to infection), low birth weight, and fetal loss
- Cerebral palsy, neonatal sepsis

Valerianna Amorosa, MD

Fever of Unknown Origin (FUO)

- An illness of greater than **3 weeks** with **fevers exceeding 101°F (38.1°C)** on repeated occasions without a diagnosis after 1 week of testing in the hospital or in an outpatient setting
- In the elderly, an increase of 2.3°F (1.3°C) from baseline temperature is considered a fever

■ Epidemiology

- Advanced laboratory, microbiologic and imaging techniques have led to earlier diagnoses of classic FUO causes
- Major diagnostic categories are **infection, connective tissue disease, and malignancy**

■ History

- Fever and associated symptoms
  - Onset, chronicity
  - Pattern: Occasionally points to diagnosis
  - Cyclic fever (e.g., malaria)
  - Relapsing fever (e.g., *Borrelia* spp: 2–3 days fever, 7–9 day afebrile interval)
  - Recurrences with afebrile periods (e.g., Still's disease, Crohn's disease, hereditary fever syndromes, Behçet's disease)
  - Response to past therapeutic trials of antibiotics, anti-inflammatory medications can be a clue
  - Patients can record pattern, associated symptoms in a **fever log**
- Past medical history
  - Age, illnesses, infections, malignancies and other immunocompromising conditions, **surgeries** and other invasive procedures
  - Implantation of **prosthetic devices** (e.g., artificial joints, pacemakers)
  - **Blood transfusions**
  - Vaccinations
- Exposure history
  - Sick contacts (e.g., Epstein-Barr virus [EBV], cytomegalovirus [CMV])
  - Detailed sexual history (e.g., HIV, syphilis)

- Lifetime tuberculosis (TB) contacts
- Details of occupational and recreational activities
- Exposure to animals (e.g., Q fever, leptospirosis)
- Military service
- Complete, **lifetime travel history** with detailed itinerary within and outside home country (e.g., histoplasmosis, malaria, typhoid)
- Diet
  - Specifics about origin of meat, dairy products, vegetables (e.g., typhoid, brucellosis)
- Medication history
  - Detailed history including **herbal supplements** (e.g., drug fever)
  - **Immunosuppressive drug history** broadens differential diagnosis (fungi and other opportunistic pathogens)
  - Illicit drugs
- Family history
  - Prior TB and other infections
  - Autoimmune diseases
  - Malignancies
  - Febrile syndromes and **ethnic origin** (See Periodic Fever Syndromes, below)
- Complete review of systems
  - Repeatedly review to ascertain forgotten clues
  - Positive findings may serve as clues to local disease or constellation of findings suggesting systemic illnesses

■ **Physical Examination**

- Systematic and repeated; clues can be transiently present and/or evolve over time
  - View the whole body
  - Remove clothing, prosthetic limbs, dentures, all bandages
  - **Detailed examination of skin** for any rash, lesions, scars (clues for Still's disease, disseminated infection, vasculitis)
- Neurological examination
  - Subtle neurological and behavioral symptoms, peripheral neuropathy, cerebellar signs (e.g., chronic meningitis, Whipple's disease)
- **Ophthalmologic examination** can give diagnostic clues
  - External exam (e.g., TB, sarcoidosis, other granulomatous disease, rheumatoid arthritis [RA])
  - Examination of retina and its vessels (e.g., endocarditis, sarcoidosis, vasculitis)
- Cardiac examination (endocarditis, atrial myxoma)

■ **BOX 18-1   Common Tests That Can Be Useful Early in Workup of FUO**

- CBC, white cell differential; review the smear
- Routine chemistries, renal function, uric acid, creatine phosphokinase
- Liver enzymes, bilirubin, lactate dehydrogenase
- Erythrocyte sedimentation rate, C-reactive protein, ferritin
- Antinuclear antibody (ANA)
- Rheumatoid factor
- Rapid plasma reagent
- Three anaerobic and aerobic sets of routine blood cultures off antibiotics
- HIV antibody (qualitative viral load if considering acute infection)
- Heterophile antibodies/further EBV serologies
- Cytomegalovirus serologies/culture of blood, urine, or other sites
- Angiotensin-converting enzyme level
- Feces for occult blood
- Urine culture, sputum culture, feces culture when indicated
- Chest x-ray
- Abdominal computed tomography (CT)
- Purified protein derivative
- Urinary histoplasmosis antigen (if any possible exposure)
- Mammogram in women
- Other age-appropriate cancer screening such as colonoscopy

Adapted from Amorosa, V. Fever of unknown origin. In: Lo Re V, ed. Hot Topics in Infectious Diseases. Philadelphia: Hanley and Belfus, 2004

- Liver and spleen
  - Assess size and texture (malignancy, disseminated infection such as EBV, histoplasmosis) and presence of **surgical scars** (history of splenectomy)
- Thorough genital and rectal examinations
  - Ulcers, masses, tenderness (sexually transmitted disease, prostatitis, malignancy, abscess, granulomatous disease, vasculitis)
- Musculoskeletal examination (e.g., occult gout, RA)

■ **Additional Studies**

- First basic laboratory studies before elaborate serologies and biologic markers (Box 18-1) (e.g., complete blood count [CBC] yielding cytopenias, atypical lymphocytosis, eosinophilia)

Microbiology
- Blood cultures
- Standard techniques can culture common causes of intravascular infections and many rarer causes (e.g., staphylococci, streptococci, HACEK organisms)
- Repeat cultures increase sensitivity
- In setting of potential exposures, specific culturing techniques are employed (e.g., **nutritional variant streptococci,** *Mycobacteria, Legionella*)
- Discuss potential organisms with microbiologist

Serologic Tests
- If exposure history or clinical clues point to viral infection, often **serology and PCR** can clarify diagnosis (e.g., EBV, HIV, CMV, parvovirus, hepatitis A and B, hepatitis C with cryoglobulinemia)
- Useful for difficult to culture bacterial pathogens; acute and convalescent serologies are often needed (e.g., *Bartonella* spp, *Borrelia* spp, *Chlamydia* spp, *Coxiella burnetii*, histoplasmosis)
- History and physical findings guide serologic testing for lupus, RA, other connective tissue and vasculitic diseases (e.g., ANA, rheumatoid factor, p-ANCA)

Radiologic Tests
- Chest X-ray
- Cross-sectional imaging (CT)
  - Can lead to diagnosis of abscess and other masses, lymphadenopathy, organomegaly
  - Can guide invasive diagnostic tests
- Other studies to consider include echocardiogram, vascular ultrasound, magnetic resonance imaging (MRI) scan, tagged white cell scans, and other nuclear imaging tests

Other Studies
- Should generally be guided by clues and become more useful when noninvasive tests not definitive (e.g., abdominal symptoms and weight loss warrant colonoscopy for inflammatory bowel disease)
- When no clues gleaned, occasionally blind biopsy can be useful
  - Data support liver biopsy for staining, exhaustive culturing in this setting (e.g., extrapulmonary TB)
  - In elderly, **temporal biopsy** may be useful (temporal arteritis)
  - Bone marrow and lymph node biopsy can also be diagnostic in certain conditions

■ **Management**
- Examine all primary data **repeatedly**
- **Revisit** history and physical examination

- Review imaging with radiologist
- Review **blood smears**
- When clues point in illogical directions, begin to **consider factitious fever**
- In cases in which exhaustive evaluation is not fruitful, further consultation with subspecialists warranted
- State of patient will dictate further management
- Empiric therapeutic trials appropriate in a deteriorating patient
- Watchful waiting with symptom management appropriate in stable patient
- Some patients will eventually be diagnosed, others will have symptom resolution, and fewer will progress

Hereditary Periodic Fever Syndromes

- Syndromes characterized by intermittent bouts of fever and inflammation with focal organ involvement. Precipitants for bouts not well characterized
- Several **genetic syndromes** have been described
- Three best-characterized diseases are **familial Mediterranean fever (FMF), familial hibernian fever** (also known as tumor necrosis factor receptor-associated periodic syndrome, **TRAPS**), and **hyperimmunoglobulinemia D (Hyper-IgD)**

■ Epidemiology

- Rare. Likelihood is determined by ethnic origin
- FMF
  - Most common periodic fever syndrome
  - **Non-Ashkenazi Jews, Turks, and Arabs** from the East most commonly, but also Arabs from the West, Armenians, Druzes, Lebanese, Italians, and Greeks
- TRAPS: Originally described in **Irish** and Nordic populations. Seen also in African-American, Japanese, and Mediterranean populations
- Hyper-IgD: Seen in **Dutch** and French

■ Etiology and Pathogenesis

- FMF: Defect in MEFV gene
  - Autosomal recessive
  - MEFV gene encodes a protein expressed in myeloid cells and involved in cytokine expression and cellular apoptosis
  - Precise mechanisms behind the role of this defect in producing inflammatory attacks are still being elucidated

- TRAPS: Defect in tumor necrosis factor (TNF) receptor super-family type 1A gene
  - Autosomal dominant with incomplete penetrance
  - Due to low concentration or dysfunction of soluble TNF receptor, there is decreased ability to neutralize action of soluble TNF-α and its downstream proinflammatory cascade
- Hyper-IgD: Involves mevalonate kinase gene
  - Autosomal recessive
  - Enzymatic disease due to relative decrease in mevalonate kinase
  - Downstream effect is increased production of specific cytokines

■ History/Physical Exam

- FMF
  - Bouts begin typically **before age 5**
  - Attacks of constant fever that can last for **hours to 3–4 days**
  - Fever associated with **abdominal pain** (peritonitis) but also large **joint synovitis** and rarely other foci of inflammation
  - **Erysipelas-like rash** of lower extremities can be seen
- TRAPS
  - **Variable age** of onset; generally diagnosed in adulthood
  - Bouts generally longer than with FMF **(5 days to weeks)**
  - Painful **myalgia** due to fascial inflammation
  - Severe **abdominal pain**
  - Rashes are common, typically "pseudocellulitis" of extremities
- Hyper-IgD
  - Symptoms often begin **first year of life**
  - Attacks average **7 days** with 4–8 weeks between
  - Can be associated with abdominal pain, diarrhea, arthritis, rash, cervical lymphadenopathy

■ Additional Studies

- White blood count, sedimentation rate, and C-reactive protein generally elevated during attack
- For FMF, TRAPS: Genetic testing with ethnicity and family history as a guide
- For Hyper-IgD: Measuring level of **mevalonate in urine** during an attack or measuring level in lymphocytes. IgD level generally elevated, although not specific

■ Differential Diagnosis

- Still's disease, inflammatory bowel disease, Behçet's disease, other autoimmune diseases can cause recurrent febrile episodes over many years

■ **Management**
- FMF: **Colchicine** to prevent recurrent attacks and the long-term sequelae of amyloidosis
- TRAPS: **Corticosteroids, etanercept**
- Hyper-IgD: Early results suggest **etanercept** may be helpful

■ **Complications**
- If FMF and TRAPS are not diagnosed and treated appropriately, amyloidosis due to chronic inflammation can occur. It has not been reported with Hyper-IgD syndrome

Tick-Borne Illnesses

Given continued human encroachment on the wilderness habitats of their natural vertebrate vectors, tick-borne diseases are continuing to emerge in humans with geographical distributions and epidemiology in constant flux

■ **Epidemiology**
- Ticks: Disease epidemiology is determined by the geographic distribution of the tick vectors that feed on humans as opportunistic hosts
- *Ixodes* ticks
  - Tiny nymph stage also transmits disease during blood meal; many patients do not report tick bite history
  - Requires at least **24 hours attachment** to transmit disease during blood meal
- *Dermacentor* ticks (dog and wood ticks)
  - Larger and more quick to transmit infection during blood meal
  - Most patients will give a tick bite history
- Other species
  - *Amblyomma americanum* (lone star tick)
  - *Ornithodoros hermsi:* Very **short attachment** required to transmit relapsing fever

■ **Diseases** (see Table 18-1 for geographic distribution)

Lyme Disease
- Over 20,000 cases reported to CDC each year
- Most commonly seen May through August
- Serologic surveillance suggests exposure to both Lyme and RMSF is widespread

Rocky Mountain Spotted Fever
- The tick-borne illness associated with the **highest fatality rate** in the US (3% to 5% when treated, up to 40% in preantibiotic era)

■ TABLE 18-1   Organisms, Associated Vectors, and North American Geographic Distribution

Disease	Organism	Known Geographic Distribution	Tick Carrier	Incubation Period
Lyme disease	Borrelia burgdorferi	Eastern, North Central, far western US	Ixodes spp	7–14 days but variable
RMSF	Rickettsia rickettsii, R. parkeri	Concentrated Southeast, seen in all states but Maine and Vermont	Dermacentor variabilis, D. andersoni	2–14 days
HME	Ehrlichia chaffeensis	Mainly Southeast, South Central and Northeast	Amblyomma americanum, D. variabilis	About 7 days
HGE	Anaplasma phagocytophila	Northeast, North Central	I. scapularis, D. variabilis	About 7 days
Babesiosis	Babesia microti	New England, mid-Atlantic states	Ixodes spp (nymphs most often)	1–8 weeks
Tularemia	Francisella tularensis	Mainly in Midwest but reported throughout US	Several species known to transmit	2–5 days (up to 25 days)
CTF	Colorado tick bite fever virus	Rocky Mountains and North to Canada	D. andersoni	1–14 days (3–4 days median)
Tick-borne relapsing fever	Borrelia hermsii	Western US, British Columbia	Ornithodoros hermsi	4–18 days

Abbreviations: CTF, Colorado tick fever; HGE, human granulocytic ehrlichiosis; HME, human monocytic ehrlichiosis; RMSF, Rocky Mountain spotted fever

- Most common April through October
- Less than 1000 cases reported to CDC per year. Likely underreported

Ehrlichiosis
- Geography of HME and HGE overlap (see Table 18-1)
- Seen generally April through October
- Less than 1000 cases reported per year, but increasing prevalence noted

Colorado Tick Fever
- Several hundred cases per year
- March through September with peak from **April to June**

Tularemia
- See Chapter 20

Others
- Other *Borrelia* and *Rickettsia* spp have been found to cause tick-borne illnesses regionally (e.g., *B. lonestari* in the South causing Lyme-like illness)
- *B. hermsii* in Western US causing relapsing fever
- Throughout the world, different ticks serve as vectors for many different illnesses. Hundreds of other *Rickettsia*, *Borrelia*, and viral tick-borne diseases can cause disease in international travelers with history of traveling to specific regions (e.g., African tick bite fever caused by *Rickettsia africae*, Mediterranean spotted fever caused by *R. conorii*)

■ Risk Factors
- Geography, time of year, and exposure to infected ticks determine risk
- Risk factors for severe disease
  - Delay in diagnosis and missed diagnosis
  - Host-related immune factors (e.g., **asplenia** and advanced age with babesiosis leads to more fulminant or prolonged course. G6PD-deficiency with RMSF associated with more severe disease)

■ Etiology

Lyme Disease
- *Borrelia burgdorferi:* Spirochete is agent of Lyme
- Coinfection of Lyme with *Babesia* or *Ehrlichia* is common

Rocky Mountain Spotted Fever
- *R. rickettsii, R. parkeri*
- Fastidious pleomorphic gram-negative rods, obligate intracellular bacteria multiply in the **cytoplasm** of infected cells

Ehrlichiosis
- *A. phagocytophila:* Tiny gram-negative organisms that cause HGE
- *E. chaffeensis*: Primary species of HME
- Other species associated with disease (e.g., *E. ewingii*)

Babesiosis
- *B. microti*, an **intracellular protozoan**, is the main species of human disease in US

Colorado Tick Fever
- CTF virus is an orbivirus **infecting marrow red cell precursors,** leading to viremia

■ **Pathogenesis**

Lyme Disease
- *Borrelia* spirochete replicates locally, then disseminates through the body
- Causes infection by migration through tissues, adhesion to host cells, and evasion of immune clearance
- Disease can manifest in several organs of the body (e.g., skin, joints, central nervous system [CNS], heart, eye)

Rocky Mountain Spotted Fever
- Organisms **invade endothelial** and other smooth muscle cells in organs throughout the body
- Leads to dermatoses, thrombocytopenia, and disseminated intravascular coagulation

Ehrlichiosis
- Infection of **white blood cells**
- HGE organisms grow within cytoplasmic vacuoles of granulocytes (morulae), leading to cytopenias and systemic symptoms

Babesiosis
- Tick introduces the sporozoite into blood. Sporozoite enters erythrocyte and multiplies in the blood, leading to systemic symptoms and hemolysis

Colorado Tick Fever
- Viremia leads to systemic symptoms

■ **History/Physical Exam**

Lyme Disease
- Tick exposure history
- With tiny nymphs, no history may be present
- **Erythema migrans** rash
  - Classic target lesion (**bull's eye** is pathognomonic) at **site of tick bite**
  - Can vary in color, shape
- Disseminated disease in days to weeks of inoculation, with multisystem involvement
  - Multiple erythema migrans lesions; systemic symptoms (malaise, low-grade fever)
  - Can have arthralgia or arthritis, carditis with **heart block,** neurological symptoms including meningitis and **Bell's palsy**
- Late disease in months to years: Persistent infection
  - Can have intermittent arthritis bouts, rarely chronic encephalomyelitis

- Post-Lyme syndromes: Treatment-resistant arthritis, chronic fatigue-like syndrome

Rocky Mountain Spotted Fever
- **Classic triad:** Fever, headache, and rash in a patient with a recent tick bite
- Rash may be present or absent, commonly not present early in course
- Initially discrete macules on wrist, ankles, spreading **centripetally** to **palms and soles,** moves centrally to trunk
- Over days, macules progress to papules, petechiae

Ehrlichiosis
- HGE and HME clinically same
- Almost all report tick exposure
- Mild to moderate acute febrile syndrome
- **"Spotless fever":** Typically, high fever, malaise, myalgia, arthralgia, abdominal pain, regional lymphadenopathy. Pneumonitis is seen

Babesiosis
- Chills, high fever, prostration, anorexia, and headache related to parasitemia
- Fatigue related to **hemolytic anemia**
- May be **coinfected with Lyme**

Colorado Tick Fever
- Abrupt onset of fevers, chills, headache, myalgias and weakness. 15% with rash
- Symptoms may remit and then return after 2–3 days. Full recovery can be delayed several weeks

■ Additional Studies

Lyme Disease
- Erythema migrans diagnosis is clinical
- Serologic testing
  - Likely negative in early disease
  - Enzyme-linked immunosorbent assay (ELISA) screen, then Western blot to increase specificity. Several Western blot bands on IgM Western blot in proper clinical setting consistent with recent infection
  - IgG Western blot bands suggest past infection
- Lumbar puncture if suspect neuroborreliosis

Rocky Mountain Spotted Fever
- Abnormal liver function tests (LFTs), **thrombocytopenia, hyponatremia**
- Serology: Acute and convalescent, **PCR**

Ehrlichiosis
- Abnormalities: Smear not sensitive but in **HGE morulae may be detected in granulocytes**
- Leukopenia, thrombocytopenia, atypical lymphocytes, abnormal LFTs all consistent
- Acute and convalescent serology, **whole blood PCR more commonly used**

Babesiosis
- Tests for hemolytic anemia (AST, bilirubin, LDH, haptoglobin). May or may not have microscopic hematuria
- **Blood smear:** Thin to demonstrate ring-forms of *Babesia*. May need multiple thin smears or quantitative buffy coat smear to determine a low-grade parasitemia
- Serology can be useful in low-grade parasitemia

Colorado Tick Fever
- PCR can rapidly diagnose. Serology and other diagnostic methods also available

■ Differential Diagnosis

In a febrile illness following known tick exposure, knowing the type of tick is helpful to narrow differential

Lyme Disease
- Primary target lesion: Classic appearance is diagnostic
- Disseminated disease differential: Rheumatologic disease, rickettsial illness, secondary syphilis
- Lyme Bell's palsy differential: HIV, syphilis, TB, sarcoidosis

Rocky Mountain Spotted Fever
- Early form can resemble gastroenteritis
- Differential: Meningitis, sepsis, leptospirosis, CTF, *Ehrlichia*

Ehrlichiosis
- Nonspecific symptoms of "summer flu"

Babesiosis
- **Smear can be confused with malaria.** High-grade parasitemia with fairly well clinical appearance counters that diagnosis

■ Management (Tables 18-2 and 18-3)
Lyme Disease
- Treatment can be complicated by lack of therapeutic endpoint
- Antibiotic administration mode and duration determined by stage of disease

■ **TABLE 18-2   Lyme Disease Stages and Treatment Recommendations of the Infectious Diseases Society of America**

Stage	Treatment	Alternative	Duration
Primary, local (target lesion)	Doxycycline	Amoxicillin	14–21 days
Primary, disseminated, without CNS involvement	Doxycycline	Amoxicillin	14–21 days
Lyme arthritis	Doxycycline	Amoxicillin	28 days*
Disseminated, with CNS involvement	Ceftriaxone	Penicillin G	14–28 days
Late, neuroborreliosis	Ceftriaxone	Penicillin G	14–28 days
Chronic Lyme disease or post-Lyme	No current evidence indicates that treatment is effective		

*If symptoms persist for months following treatment, another course is recommended

■ **TABLE 18-3   Selected Tick-Borne Diseases and First-Line Treatments**

Disease	Treatment
RMSF	Doxycycline
Ehrlichiosis	Doxycycline
Babesiosis	Quinine sulfate + clindamycin, or atovaquone + azithromycin
Tularemia	Streptomycin or gentamicin
CTF	Supportive, possible role for ribavirin
Tick-borne relapsing fever	Doxycycline

Abbreviations: CTF, Colorado tick fever; RMSF, Rocky Mountain spotted fever

Rocky Mountain Spotted Fever
- Early consideration and empiric treatment key to decreasing morbidity. **Higher mortality if treatment started more than 5 days after initial symptoms**
- Supportive care for organ and hematological involvement

Ehrlichiosis
- Treatment with **doxycycline** leads to rapid improvement

■ Complications
- Lyme disease: Arthropathy, chronic fatigue, or post-Lyme syndrome

- RMSF: Acute respiratory distress syndrome (ARDS), renal failure, multiorgan system failure, and death
- Ehrlichiosis: In immunocompromised patients, can present with severe manifestations
- Babesiosis: Massive hemolysis can lead to severe anemia and renal failure

19

Travel Medicine

Paul Pottinger, MD, DTM&H

Pretravel Preparation

- More than 20 million Americans travel overseas each year
- Exotic destinations are increasingly popular
- Illness is common but **often preventable**
- Most pretravel care is provided by primary care physicians, **not** travel clinics

■ General Medical Advice

- Causes of death among Americans when abroad:
  - Myocardial infarction (MI) and cerebrovascular accident 35% to 69%, trauma 21% to 26%, infection 1% to 4%
- **Plan** meticulously for patients with chronic illnesses; **ordering vaccines alone is insufficient**
- **Prescribe** extra medications and supplies (e.g., insulin syringes) for carry-on—**not checked**—luggage
- **Discuss** itinerary (transportation, activities, accommodations, food, water)
- **Warn** patients to maintain good judgment when abroad
  - Sexually transmissible disease (STD) rates (including HIV and hepatitis B) often high, especially among commercial sex workers; consider bringing condoms
  - Motor vehicle injuries linked to alcohol and no seatbelt use
  - Check for US State Department safety notices at http://travel. state.gov/
- **Document** diagnoses, medications, allergies, contact info with medical alert bracelet or letter in local language. Consider registering on arrival with local consulate or embassy (http://www. travel.state.gov)
- **Reminder:** Medical evacuation can cost over $10,000; consider medical evacuation insurance (e.g., http://www.insuremytrip.com)
- **Deep venous thrombosis (DVT)**
  - Risk increases with length of flight
  - Walk at least once per hour
- **Respiratory infections**
  - Hand hygiene critical (alcohol gels or handwashing)

- **Bring** N95 mask (filters 1-μm particles with an efficiency of at least 95%) if anticipate heavy exposure to airborne pathogens (TB, SARS, influenza), particularly if compromised host
- **Wear** mask if near coughing passengers
- Jet lag
  - Circadian rhythm adjusts one time zone per day (maximum)
  - No drug regimen defeats it (including melatonin)
  - Adapt in advance (move bedtime and wake time 1 hour per day)
- **Malaria and diarrhea prophylaxis** (see below)

■ Vaccines

- Optimum lead time is 6 months prior to departure
- Guidelines at Centers for Disease Control web page (http://www. cdc.gov/travel/vaccinat.htm)

Routine Adult Vaccination Series

- Some infections rarely seen in US are **endemic** overseas
- Many Americans not vaccinated per CDC guidelines; can check antibody titers, but slow and costly. Alternatively:
  - **Check for recent outbreaks** at http://www.cdc.gov/travel/outbreaks.htm
  - **Tetanus-diphtheria** booster offered to **everyone** after primary series every 10 years, or once if over 50 years old
  - **Influenza** transmission year-round in tropics, so offer vaccine if available (US strains may differ from tropical strains)
  - **MMR** booster offered if traveling to endemic areas (even those born before 1957) if low or unknown titers unless immunosuppressed
  - **Pneumovax:** Same indications as in nontravelers
  - **Polio** booster (injectable) offered if unclear immunity
  - **Varicella** booster if no protective Ab titers or history of infection

Cholera

- ***Vibrio cholerae*** is a gram-negative rod
- Fecal-oral spread
- Severe secretory diarrhea usually self-limited
- Endemic in much of developing world, especially India
- No vaccine available in US; Canada and Europe use oral vaccine: 85% immune for 3 months → 30% in 3 yrs
- Treatment: Rehydration

Hepatitis A

- Positive-sense RNA picornavirus
- Fecal-oral spread

- Self-limited jaundice; can progress to fulminant hepatic failure
- Endemic in most of developing world; offer vaccine to all non-immune travelers. US risk is highest in Western states
- Inactivated whole-cell vaccine: Inject day 0 and 2nd injection between months 6 and 12. Short-term immunity by week 4
- Lifelong immunity after booster; no contraindications

Hepatitis B

- DNA hepadnavirus; blood or sexual transmission
- Disease may be acute and self-limited or progress to hepatic failure or hepatocellular carcinoma
- Risk intermediate or high in all of developing world (but lower than hepatitis A); offer vaccine to nonimmune patients planning a stay of longer than 6 months or with high-risk behavior (healthcare workers, needle use, unprotected sex)
- Recombinant vaccine; several dosing schedules:
  - **Standard:** Day 0, month 6, month 12 (consider Twinrix [combined hepatitis A and B vaccine] if hepatitis A nonimmune)
  - **Accelerated:** Day 0, month 1, month 2, month 12
  - **Ultra-accelerated:** Day 0, day 7, day 21, month 12
- Immunity lifelong in 95% of patients; check titers 2 months after series only in high-risk patients; no contraindications

Japanese Encephalitis

- Flavivirus spread by mosquito; case fatality rate 30%
- Endemic and epidemic in Southeast Asia; 50,000 cases per year in natives, but only ~1 case per year in US travelers
- Offer if traveling outdoors in rural Southeast Asia
- Whole-cell inactivated vaccine: Inject day 0, 7, 30; immunity at day 40 is 70% to 97%; boost every 2 years

Meningococcus

- *Neisseria meningitidis* is a gram-negative diplococcus spread by nasal secretions and droplets
- May cause life-threatening meningitis or dissemination with shock, purpura, and cardiovascular collapse
- Risk low, but highest in crowded living situations (entering military or college, travel to Mecca or sub-Saharan "meningitis belt" during dry season) or host with asplenia or terminal complement deficiency
- Vaccine required of pilgrims making hajj in Mecca
- Quadrivalent vaccine (A, C, Y, W-135): Single injection, immune by day 14
- Immunity wanes over 3–10 years

Rabies
- Negative-sense RNA rhabdovirus
- Fatal after animal bite without postexposure prophylaxis; passive antibody administration with half of HRIG dose injected around wound, half in delfoid, plus vaccine
- Risk low; offer vaccine if working with animals or living in endemic nations longer than 4 weeks
- Inactivated whole-cell or adsorbed vaccine for **preexposure prophylaxis consists of 3 injections;** inject IM day 0, 7, and 21 or 28 (if given intradermally, must complete series 1 month before starting medications such as chloroquine [CQ] for malaria prophylaxis)
- Immunity always **partial;** allows abbreviated postexposure prophylaxis without rabies immunoglobulin

Tuberculosis (TB; see also Chapter 9)
- Latent TB in about 50% of all people, about 5% will reactivate
- Document **TB test (PPD)** pretravel and 3 months postreturn
- Use of bacille Calmette-Guérin vaccine (BCG) or recombinant BCG is controversial in travelers; not typically used in US, rarely offered to children living in highly endemic areas for longer than 6 months

Typhoid
- *Salmonella typhi* is an enteric gram-negative rod
- Fecal-oral spread
- Systemic illness with serious morbidity/mortality
- Endemic in much of developing world; risk highest in Indian subcontinent (~100 cases per million travelers) versus Southeast Asia or sub-Saharan Africa (fewer than 10 cases per million travelers). Offer vaccine to patients visiting relatives, traveling longer than 2 weeks, or backpacking
- **Preferred vaccine:** Capsular polysaccharide by single IM injection; 50% to 80% protection at week 2 for 3–5 years; no contraindications
- **Older vaccine:** Live attenuated *S. typhi* by 4 PO doses every other day, finishing 2 weeks before departure; medications such as CQ interfere; contraindicated in compromised hosts
- **Oldest vaccine:** Inactivated whole-cell, no longer used

Yellow Fever
- Positive-sense RNA flavivirus
- Mosquito-borne
- Hemorrhagic fever endemic in parts of Latin America and Africa. Risk of infection low, but incidence can approach 1 in 250 during epidemics, and mortality can reach 50%
- Live-attenuated vaccine: Inject day 0, immune day 10

- Boost every 10 years
- Proof of vaccination required for entry into some nations: Check destination at http://www.cdc.gov/travel/yb/outline. htm#2
- Vaccine safe overall: 13 encephalitis cases/100 million doses, ~100 adverse events/year. Contraindicated in AIDS, pregnancy, immunosuppression, egg allergy, age below 9 months or over 70 years

Malaria

- Curable, but potentially fatal if misdiagnosed
- Involve infectious disease service or CDC malaria hotline (1-770-488-7788)
- Emphasize "ABCDs" with patients:
  - **A**wareness of the risk, incubation period, and symptoms
  - **B**ite of the mosquito should be avoided
  - **C**hemoprophylaxis must be taken as directed
  - **D**iagnosis and treatment should be sought immediately for any fever developing beyond 1 week after entering or less than 6 months after returning from endemic areas

■ Epidemiology

- Endemic in many (but not all) tropical regions
- 200–300 million cases worldwide per year; 1–2 million deaths, most sub-Saharan African children under 5 years old
- Diagnosed in 30% to 40% of travelers admitted worldwide for fever returning from endemic areas (~30,000 cases per year)

■ Risk Factors

- Mandatory: Bite of infected female *Anopheles* mosquito
- Contributory: Nonimmune (tourists and natives returning after absence), pregnancy, immunosuppression, lack of pro-phylaxis
- Year-round transmission, but risk rises after rainy season

■ Etiology

- During mosquito's blood meal, protozoan parasites of genus *Plasmodium* injected into host
- Four species cause human disease: ***P. falciparum, P. vivax, P. ovale,*** and ***P. malariae***
- Proportion of species varies with region
- Vertical and transfusion-borne transmission also possible

■ Pathogenesis

- Sporozoites injected by mosquito into dermis, enter liver, develop into schizonts, and in 6–16 days release thousands of merozoites into bloodstream. Merozoites enter red blood cells (RBCs), multiply as "ring" trophozoites, and mature into schizonts, which pack the RBC and scavenge its heme and glucose. More merozoites are released into bloodstream and some become gametocytes, which are taken up by another mosquito to complete life cycle
- In *P. vivax* and *P. ovale* infections, some merozoites become hypnozoites, which can remain dormant for months or years
- Synchronized release of merozoites from RBCs causes cyclic fever and malaise (every 48 hours for **falciparum, vivax, and ovale;** every 72 hours for **malariae**)
- Infected RBCs adhere to vessel walls, causing sluggish end-organ blood flow and cerebral malaria and renal failure (**falciparum**)
- Anemia from hemoglobin consumption, RBC lysis, and hepatosplenic sequestration (all species)

■ Prevention

Determine risk by checking destination at http://www.cdc.gov/travel/yb/outline.htm#2. If malaria endemic:
- Mosquito avoidance
  - Most feeding happens at dusk
  - DEET, picardin, or lemon eucalyptus oil all excellent
  - Permethrin on clothing and bed nets increases protection
  - These measures also protect from other arthropod-borne diseases (e.g., dengue, viral encephalitis, filariasis, trypanosomiasis)
- Pharmacologic prophylaxis regimen depends on CQ resistance at destination (reported at CDC web site)
  - If no CQ resistance, prescribe it as first line
  - If CQ resistance, choose from:
    - **Mefloquine.** Resistance in Thailand, Cambodia, and Myanmar. Small risk of psychosis if recent mental illness
    - **Atovaquone/proguanil.** Resistance is very rare (a few case reports in Africa). Note: Costs over $5/day
    - **Doxycycline.** Resistance rare and may prevent leptospirosis. Note: Inexpensive, but risk photosensitivity, esophagitis, decreased oral contraceptive efficacy
  - In each case, take **before, during, and after** trip as directed
- If medical care will be more than 1 day away, offer stand-by emergency treatment: A 3-day supply of atovaquone/proguanil

■ **History/Physical Exam**

- Determine exposure via **itinerary, mosquito bites,** and **timing** (incubation 10 days to 6 months or more)
- **Fever mandatory,** but pattern **not always** every 48 or 72 hrs
- Malaise and fatigue **common**
- Presence of dark urine, jaundice, abdominal pain, diarrhea, shortness of breath, cough, and seizure; coma **less common**
- Determine host immune status (prophylaxis used, pregnancy, prior exposure, hemoglobinopathy)
- Look for signs of anemia (tachycardia, pallor), hemolysis (jaundice, scleral icterus), sequestration (hepatosplenomegaly)
- Look for central nervous system (CNS) dysfunction (altered mental status, seizure, diffuse upper motor neuron deficits)

■ **Additional Studies**

- **STAT peripheral blood smears are mandatory!**
- If possible, collect from finger stick directly onto slide or into red top tube, and immediately process in lab
- Thick smear: Lysed heap of RBCs (more sensitive)
- Thin smear: Intact RBC monolayer (better for species identification)
- Repeat smears every 6–12 hours and with fever spikes until malaria ruled in or alternative diagnosis made
- Antigen assays available at reference laboratories if repeat smears are negative
- Consider complete blood count (CBC) with differential, chemistry panel, urinalysis, β-HCG, and HIV; head CT, LP

■ **Differential Diagnosis**

- **Malaria always at top of differential** for patients with fever after returning from tropics!
- Also consider dengue, typhoid, acute HIV, respiratory or GI viral infection, meningitis (see Fever in the Returning Traveler, below)
- Note: **Malaria often a coinfection;** if no improvement with treatment of another infection, consider undiagnosed malaria

■ **Management**

Determine species as soon as possible:
- If non-falciparum:
  - Often manage as outpatient unless significant comorbidity
  - Prescribe oral CQ for 3 days, then oral primaquine for 2 weeks if *P. vivax* or *P. ovale* (kill hypnozoites)
- If falciparum:

- Low threshold to hospitalize until clinical response assured
- Prescribe quinine or quinidine, plus doxycycline or clindamycin for 7 days. Watch for hypoglycemia, long QT changes, cinchonism (reversible tinnitus and high-tone deafness)
- Daily parasitemia counts
- Meticulous supportive care for **complicated malaria:** Cerebral malaria, severe anemia, renal failure, cardiopulmonary distress

■ Complications

- Poor outcomes with **late presentation** or **missed diagnosis**
- Untreated falciparum malaria is **often fatal**
- Treated severe falciparum: CNS deficits, disseminated intravascular coagulation (DIC), acute respiratory distress syndrome (ARDS), acute renal failure
- *P. vivax* and *P. ovale* infections may "relapse" due to hypnozoites, rarely cause massive hepatosplenomegaly
- *P. malariae* can cause nephritis

Traveler's Diarrhea and Intestinal Parasites

- Affects over 30% of travelers to Southeast Asia, Africa, India, and Latin America
- Food/water-borne infections (bacteria, viruses, fungi, parasites)

■ Prevention

- Educate: Fecal-oral transmission ("boil it, cook it, peel it, or forget it"; carbonated beverages safer; filter or treat water; hand hygiene)
- Suggest: Bismuth subsalicylate 2 tabs PO four times daily to cut risk by 60% (note: constipating; avoid salicylate intoxication if on aspirin, methotrexate, warfarin, probenecid, or travel for longer than 3 weeks)
- Not recommended: Prophylactic antibiotics
  - Rifaximin prophylaxis likely safe, but limited efficacy data preclude routine use

■ Clinical Manifestations

- **Bland diarrhea most common:** Little fever or cramping, watery stool, normal white blood cells (WBCs), nontoxic overall appearance
  - Causes often enterotoxic *Escherichia coli*, *Bacillus cereus*, *Staphylococcus aureus*, *Giardia*, viruses, etc.
  - Treatment: Hydration, BRAT diet (bananas, rice, applesauce, toast); reevaluate if symptoms worsen or persist longer than 7 days

- **Inflammatory diarrhea (dysentery) less common:** Fever, abdominal pain, purulent/bloody stools, elevated WBC levels, toxic
  - Causes include *Campylobacter,* non-*typhi Salmonella,* enterohemorrhagic *E. coli, Shigella, Entamoeba histolytica, Clostridium difficile*
  - Treatment: Hydration, BRAT diet, check stool studies (WBCs, culture and sensitivity, ova and parasites [O&P], *C. difficile* studies); consider empiric fluoroquinolone if compromised host or severely ill

Classic Intestinal Parasite Pearls

- **Ascaris:** Roundworm; passes per rectum; often asymptomatic, can trigger appendicitis or migrate into biliary tree or peritoneum. Diagnosis: O&P. Prescribe albendazole ± pyrantel pamoate
- **Entamoeba histolytica:** Bloody diarrhea refractory to quinolones. Diagnosis: Steaming-fresh stool wet mount and O&P. Prescribe metronidazole
- **Enterobius:** Pinworm; pruritic nocturnal perianal lesions in childcare workers. Diagnosis: scotch tape prep of perianal skin. Prescribe albendazole
- **Giardia:** Watery diarrhea and upper GI upset, belching, and/or reflux after hiking or urban travel (especially Russia). Diagnosis: stool antigen. Prescribe metronidazole
- **Necator** and **Ancylostoma:** Hookworms; diarrhea, anemia, growth restriction in children after pruritic lower extremity rash at entry site. Diagnosis: Eosinophilia and O&P. Prescribe mebendazole
- **Strongyloides:** Autoinfection can cause longstanding diarrhea or subclinical infection; immunosuppression can trigger hyperinfection dissemination many years later. Diagnosis: O&P and/or serum Ag. Prescribe ivermectin
- **Taenia:** Tapeworms; flat, white proglottids about the size of a fingernail are seen in stool. Motile with asymptomatic *T. saginata* (beef) infection. Nonmotile with *T. solium* (pork) worm which can cause cysticercosis, and with less-symptomatic *T. latum* (fish) worm. Diagnosis: O&P. Prescribe albendazole
- **Trichuris:** Whipworm; mucopurulent stools and rectal prolapse. Diagnosis: O&P. Prescribe mebendazole

Fever in the Returning Traveler

- For every 100,000 travelers to developing world for more than 1 month, 50,000 fall ill, 8000 seek medical help, 5000 are bedridden, 300 are admitted, and one dies

■ **TABLE 19-1** Tropical Exposure and Major Differential Diagnosis for Fever Lasting More Than 1 Week

Exposure	Infection or Disease
Exotic foods, untreated water	Enteric infections, trichinosis, amoebiasis, hepatitis A
Unpasteurized dairy products	Brucellosis, TB
Swimming in fresh water	Leptospirosis, naegleriosis, schistosomiasis, melioidosis
Sexual contact	HIV, syphilis, gonorrhea, chancroid, hepatitis B, chlamydia
Exposure to infected person	Meningococcemia, hepatitis A, typhoid, VHF, TB, SARS, flu
Animal exposure or bite	Rabies, Q fever, tularemia, borreliosis, VHF, plague
Insect bite	**Mosquito:** Malaria, dengue, lymphatic filariasis, yellow fever
	Tick: Typhus, tularemia, borelliosis, relapsing fever, rickettsiae
	Reduviid bug: Chagas' disease
	Sand fly: Leishmaniasis
	Tsetse fly: African trypanosomiasis (sleeping sickness)
	Tumbu fly: Myiasis (various fly larvae, including bot fly)
	Louse: Plague, typhus, relapsing fever
	Mite: Scrub typhus
	Flea: Plague, *Tunga penetrans* (jiggers)

Adapted from: Humar A, Keystone J. Evaluating fever in travellers returning from tropical countries. Brit Med J 1996;312:953–956.

- Broad differential for fever lasting over 1 week, however:
  - Malaria is single most common cause (see above)
  - Always consider malaria, typhoid, and dengue fever
  - Infections common in US are also common abroad
  - Careful history and physical with standard lab tests often lead to diagnosis

■ **History**

- Detailed itinerary: Mode of travel, season, accommodations, food and drink, activities, prophylaxis, exposures (sex, insect bites, ill contacts; Table 19-1)
- Timing of symptoms: Narrows differential (Box 19-1)

■ **Physical Exam**

- Malaise: Nonspecific
- Jaundice/icterus: Hepatitis or hemolysis (malaria)

■ **BOX 19-1   Typical Incubation Periods for Selected Tropical Infections**

Short (<10 days)
Arbovirus (dengue)

Enteric fever

Influenza

Plague

Rickettsiae

Typhoid

Severe acute respiratory syndrome (SARS)

Viral hemorrhagic fever (Lassa, Ebola, Marburg)

Medium (10–21 days)
Malaria

Brucellosis

Leptospirosis

Q fever

Scrub typhus

Spotted fevers

Trypanosomiasis

Typhoid

Long (>21 days)
Malaria

Amebic abscess

Filariasis

HIV

Leishmaniasis

Viral hepatitis

Schistosomiasis

TB

Adapted from: Strickland GT, et al, eds. Hunter's Tropical Medicine. 8th Ed. Philadelphia: WB Saunders, 1997.

- Eschar: Borreliosis, typhus
- Petechiae or hemorrhage: Viral hemorrhagic fever (VHF), Rocky Mountain spotted fever, pertussis, meningococcemia
- Erythematous rash: Viral exanthem, drug fever
- Lymphadenopathy: Acute viral infection (HIV, flu, mononucleosis, dengue), rickettsiae, African trypanosomiasis, plague

- Hepatosplenomegaly: Malaria, dengue, typhoid, hepatitis, leptospirosis, ameboma, visceral leishmaniasis, relapsing fever, hydatid cyst
- CNS findings: Meningitis, hydatid cyst, neurocysticercosis

■ Additional Studies

- Thick and thin blood smears for malaria, repeated every 6–12 hours and with fevers, until diagnosis confirmed or another diagnosis made
- Blood cultures, CBC with differential (quantify eosinophils), chemistry panel with LFTs, HIV test
- Freeze a red top tube (may need "acute" serologies later)
- As indicated: Urinalysis with culture and sensitivity, stool WBC, O&P, and culture and sensitivity; chest x-ray and other imaging

■ Management

- Whenever possible, delay antimicrobial therapy until diagnosis
- Admission and empiric treatment are indicated for unstable patients; if initial workup unclear or pending, cover malaria or other likely infection (meningitis, bacteremia, pneumonia)
- Low threshold to contact infectious disease service early in workup

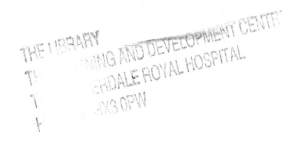

20
Biowarfare Agents

Maureen Chase, MD and Worth W. Everett, MD

- Biowarfare is now an inevitable concern for physicians
- The organisms discussed in this chapter are ideal weapons of terrorism, because they are highly stable, relatively easy to disperse (typically in aerosolized form), require a short incubation period, and are capable of causing widespread, devastating disease
- An elevated index of suspicion must be maintained, since delays in the diagnosis and treatment of intentional infections can lead to increased mortality. Suspicious presentations, clustering of unusual cases, and resistance to therapies should raise concerns for possible infection by these organisms
- Specialized testing is available through local and state public health departments
  - Meticulous containment/isolation measures should be taken until the disease(s) are known
  - Common findings, diagnostic evaluation, and treatments are summarized in Table 20-1

Anthrax

Bacillus anthracis is an aerobic, spore-forming bacterium found worldwide in the soil

■ Epidemiology/Risk Factors

- **No human-to-human transmission**
- Infection typically results from occupational exposure to sick animals (especially cattle and sheep) and their products such as wool (wool sorter's disease), meat, and skin
- Detection requires a high index of suspicion in patients lacking typical occupational exposures
- Mortality dependent on the form of anthrax infection
  - Cutaneous (most common): Untreated, 20% mortality; less than 1% if treated
  - Inhalational: Over 90% mortality whether treated or untreated
  - Gastrointestinal: Mortality is 25% to 60% despite treatment

■ **TABLE 20-1 Inhalational Presentations of Biowarfare Agents**

Agent	Classic Findings	Studies	Treatment
Anthrax	Severe respiratory illness	GS: Rod with central spore; CXR: hemorrhagic mediastinitis	Ciprofloxacin or doxycycline + one or two additional antibiotics + anthrax vaccine
Plague	Buboes; Severe pneumonia and hemoptysis	GS: Safety-pin or bipolar staining; CXR: multilobar pneumonia	Gentamicin or streptomycin; Strict respiratory droplet precautions; No vaccine
Smallpox	Vesiculopapular rash on face, hands; All lesions in same stage	Electron microscopy of vesicle fluid	Supportive care; Quarantine; Vaccinate within 72 hours
Tularemia	Generalized myalgias, HA, leading to severe bronchopneumonia	CXR: Multilobar pneumonia, hilar LAD, and pleural effusions	Streptomycin or gentamicin

Abbreviations: GS, Gram stain; HA, headache; LAD, lymphadenopathy; CXR, chest radiograph

■ **Etiology**
- *B. anthracis* is a nonmotile gram-positive rod with a centrally located spore

■ **Pathogenesis**
- Spores are inhaled, ingested, or inoculated into skin
- Virulence related to polysaccharide capsule and anthrax toxin
  - Capsule prevents phagocytosis
  - Toxin is composed of three proteins (protective antigen, edema factor, and lethal factor) that act synergistically to lyse cells and evoke an inflammatory response

■ **History/Physical Exam**
Cutaneous Anthrax
Painless, pruritic papule develops 1–14 days after inoculation of anthrax spores into skin, toxin production causes extensive edema and vesicles to form at the site, and vesicles rupture, resulting in ulceration with development of characteristic **painless black eschar** and enlarged local lymph nodes

Inhalational Anthrax

- Inhaled anthrax spores ingested by alveolar macrophages, transported to hilar lymph nodes, and germinate, releasing large amounts of toxin that causes localized edema and hemorrhage
- Several days of a flu-like illness with a nonproductive cough, myalgias, and malaise followed by acute onset of respiratory distress, fever
- Early in illness, findings consistent with a viral respiratory illness
- Later in infection patients appear acutely ill with dyspnea, cyanosis, tachycardia, diaphoresis, and fever
- **Hemorrhagic mediastinitis** is the hallmark finding
- Chest x-ray (CXR): Widened mediastinum, pleural effusions, and infiltrates
- Chest CT: Hemorrhagic mediastinal lymphadenopathy, edema, peribronchial thickening, and effusions

Gastrointestinal Anthrax

- Occurs within days of ingestion of infected or contaminated meat
- Causes ulceration of oropharyngeal and esophageal mucosa with intestinal edema, adenitis, and hemorrhage
- Presents as severe gastroenteritis with dysphagia, severe abdominal pain, fever, and bloody diarrhea
- May progress to toxemia, shock, and death

■ Additional Studies

- Blood and vesicle samples may yield presumptive diagnosis based on Gram stain appearance of nonmotile rods with a centrally located spore, which form classic encapsulated chains (bamboo rods)
- Gray, irregularly shaped colonies grow without hemolysis on sheep blood agar
- Sputum and stool cultures rarely yield positive cultures
- Nasal swabs may be performed for testing through state health department labs
- **Anthrax toxin antibody blood test** for rapid (less than 4 hour) diagnosis approved in June 2004

■ Differential Diagnosis

- Cutaneous: Insect bites, spider bites, tularemia, or ecthyma gangrenosum
- Inhalational: Influenza, histoplasmosis, sarcoid, tuberculosis (TB), or lymphoma

- Gastrointestinal: Other infectious causes of hemorrhagic enteritis including *Salmonella*, *Escherichia coli*, or *Shigella*

■ Management

- **Initial therapy with ciprofloxacin or doxycycline with one or two additional antibiotics improves survival** (potential additional antibiotics include penicillin, ampicillin, rifampin, imipenem, vancomycin, clindamycin, and clarithromycin)
- Parenteral therapy should continue until patient is stable, then oral antibiotics continued for at least 60 days
- Oral therapy (60 days) for patients exposed to a common source without signs of active disease include ciprofloxacin, doxycycline, or amoxicillin
- Standard isolation precautions are sufficient. There is no need for airborne precautions, as there is no human-to-human transmission and therefore no need to treat close contacts unless they also had exposure to the source
- Anthrax vaccine available in limited supply and recommended for veterinarians, farm workers, military, laboratory personnel working with anthrax, and patients with anthrax exposure

■ Complications

- Hemorrhagic meningitis and sepsis are almost always fatal
- Renal and ophthalmologic anthrax are rare

Plague

Enzootic infection of rodents by *Yersinia pestis*

■ Epidemiology

- Responsible for the deaths of an estimated one third of the European population in the fourteenth century (bubonic plague or "Black Death")
- **Humans infected through bites from plague-infected fleas** or, less commonly, from contact with infected animals
- 10–15 cases occur naturally in the US each year in the Pacific and Southwest regions
- Mortality depends on the form of plague:
  - Bubonic: Up to 60% mortality if untreated, 15% if treated
  - Septicemic: 30% if treated, 100% if untreated
  - Pneumonic: Nearly 100% if not treated promptly

■ Risk Factors

- Occupational exposure, living in endemic region, close (less than 2 m) contact with infected person

■ Etiology

- *Y. pestis*, a gram-negative, intracellular, facultatively anaerobic bacterium, has a characteristic bipolar or "safety pin" appearance on Wright's–Giemsa staining

■ Pathogenesis

- *Yersinia* outer proteins (Yops) block phagocytosis of the bacteria, allowing for rapid multiplication in the extracellular space of lymphoid tissues (buboes). Dissemination results in hematogenous spread and septicemia
- Similar process occurs in the lungs in pneumonic plague after inhalation of aerosolized bacteria
- Three clinical forms of the disease:
  - Bubonic plague: **Most common form** seen as an acute febrile illness with enlarged lymph nodes
  - Septicemic plague: Gram-negative sepsis in absence of buboes
  - Pneumonic plague: **Person-to-person transmission** by respiratory droplets. Likely presentation of illness if aerosolized as biowarfare agent

■ History/Physical Exam

- **Incubation period ranges from 1 to 6 days**
- Patients present with an acute febrile illness, malaise, weakness, gastrointestinal symptoms ± buboes
- Bubonic plague: An acute febrile illness with swollen, tender lymphadenopathy (buboes) in groin, axilla, and cervical regions
- Pneumonic plague:
  - Patients appear acutely ill with fever > 101.3°F (38.5°C)
  - Productive cough of watery sputum
  - **Hemoptysis** frequently occurs, ± tachypnea and hypoxia
  - Pulmonary exam consistent with severe pneumonia
  - Patients have rapid clinical deterioration within 24–28 hours to respiratory failure, sepsis, and death if unrecognized
  - CXR shows patchy **multilobar consolidation and alveolar hemorrhage**
- Consider the diagnosis when multiple patients have multilobar pneumonias unresponsive to routine antibiotics used for community-acquired pneumonia (CAP)

■ Additional Studies

- *Y. pestis* can be isolated from blood and sputum cultures and bubo aspirates
- Neutrophil predominant leukocytosis, rare leukemoid reactions and disseminated intravascular coagulation (DIC)

- Immunofluorescence antibody (sensitivity 52% to 100%, specificity 100%) and ELISA (sensitivity 90% to 100%, specificity 98% to 100%) tests available

■ Differential Diagnosis

- Infectious causes of lymphadenopathy, including cat-scratch disease, and severe CAPs (*Mycoplasma*, *Chlamydia*, *Streptococcus pneumoniae*)
- Reliance on automated microbiology testing units alone is not advised because misidentification as *Y. pseudotuberculosis*, a more common form of *Yersinia*, may occur. When *Y. pestis* is suspected, a combination of blood, sputum, and lymph cultures, as well as specialized immunostaining and polymerase chain reaction testing is recommended. They may only be available through state or federal health departments

■ Management

- First-line therapy: Gentamicin or streptomycin
- Second-line therapy: Doxycycline, fluoroquinolones, and chloramphenicol
- Strict respiratory droplet isolation precautions for at least 48 hours of antibiotic therapy
- Oral prophylaxis for close (less than 2 m) contacts with doxycycline or ciprofloxacin for 7 days. Second line oral prophylaxis agent is chloramphenicol

■ Complications

- Bactericidal antibiotic therapy may precipitate endotoxic shock
- Other complications include meningitis, endophthalmitis, DIC, and acute respiratory distress syndrome (ARDS)
- Vaccine no longer available but was ineffective against the pneumonic form of the disease

Smallpox

Smallpox was a naturally occurring disease caused by the variola virus, a member of the poxvirus family that includes monkeypox and vaccinia (smallpox vaccine)

■ Epidemiology

- Last naturally occurring case occurred in Somalia in 1977
- Disease declared eradicated by the WHO in 1980
- Only known stockpiles were in government research labs
- Ideal as a biological warfare agent due to largely nonimmunized worldwide population
- Humans are the only known reservoir

■ Risk Factors

- Historically, infection occurred from close contact with respiratory secretions or less commonly by contact with linens or clothing of an infected person
- Close contact with an infected person with characteristic rash. Greatest infectivity early in rash stage
- Any new smallpox case now considered bioterrorism

■ Etiology

- Variola virus: Double-stranded DNA virus shaped like bricks on electron micrographs
- There are two strains of the variola virus:
  - Variola major: Typical form with mortality of 30%
  - Variola minor (alastrim): Milder form with mortality 1%

■ Pathogenesis

- Virus inhaled and absorbed in mucosa
- Asymptomatic 7–17-day incubation period
- Virus migrates to regional lymph nodes for replication, then to spleen, bone marrow, and systemic lymph nodes
- Death thought to result from circulating immune complexes, which typically occur during second week of illness

■ History/Physical Exam

- Abrupt onset of severe febrile illness with headache, myalgias, rigors, and vomiting
- Oropharyngeal ulcerative lesions appear early in course
- Maculopapular **rash starts 2–3 days later on extremities and face** (most dense on face and arms)
- **Rash spreads centripetally** and progresses to vesicles (day 3); deep, tense pustules (day 5); then to crusted scabs (day 8)
- Characteristic rash with **all lesions in the same stage of development**

■ Additional Studies

- Cotton swab sample of vesicle or pustule fluid for electron microscopy
- Rapid PCR available from Centers for Disease Control (CDC) and US Army

■ Differential Diagnosis

- Varicella
  - Rash starts on trunk and spreads outward, rarely involves palms and soles; pustules are superficial
  - Lesions vary in stage of development

- Bullous impetigo, disseminated herpes zoster, drug eruptions, and other disseminated viral exanthems

■ **Management**
- Supportive care; no definitive treatment
- Patients should be isolated in negative-pressure rooms with both contact and respiratory precautions, and quarantined until all lesions have dried up
- Vaccination with live vaccinia virus within 72 hours of exposure decreases severity of disease and confers immunity for at least 5 years
- Recent military prophylactic vaccination experience resulted in local vaccinia rashes and new cases of myopericarditis
- Close contacts and health care workers should be vaccinated. Quarantine only needed if fever develops

■ **Complications**
- Blindness
- Hemorrhagic complications such as DIC, secondary bacterial infections, encephalitis, and pulmonary edema
- High mortality if unvaccinated

Tularemia

- *Francisella tularensis* is the causative bacterial agent of tularemia, also known as "deer fly fever" and "rabbit fever"
- The organism is both highly infectious and hardy, making it an ideal aerosolized biowarfare agent
- There are several disease states depending upon mode of exposure: Ulceroglandular, oculoglandular, oropharyngeal/gastrointestinal, typhoidal, and pneumonic

■ **Epidemiology**
- *F. tularensis* is endemic in the US and in Europe
- Reservoirs: Rabbits, hare, deer, squirrels, muskrats, and cats
- Vectors: Ticks, mosquitoes, and biting flies
- There is no human-to-human transmission
- Mortality when treated approaches 1%. Untreated pneumonic form is highly fatal, approaching 40%. Untreated typhoidal form has a mortality of approximately 20%

■ **Risk Factors**
- Humans are naturally exposed by bites of infected arthropods, direct contact with infected tissues (hunters, trappers), ingestion of contaminated food and water, or by inhalation of the organisms

- Occupational or accidental infection in individual cases, aerosolized exposure in widespread disease

■ Etiology

- *F. tularensis* is a gram-negative intracellular coccobacillus that requires cystine-supplemented agar for growth, making identification otherwise difficult
- **Small inoculum (10–50 organisms) can cause disease**

■ Pathogenesis

- *F. tularensis* has a thin polysaccharide capsule that allows it to remain virulent for months on animal carcasses
- Bacteria survive phagocytosis in macrophages, where they multiply, and then migrate to the regional lymph nodes, spleen, lungs and pleura, spleen, and liver
- **Necrotizing granulomas** develop that destroy tissues
- Further dissemination of bacteria can result in septic shock, organ system failure, ARDS, DIC, and death

■ History/Physical Exam

- Varies with form of disease:
  - **Ulceroglandular** (most common): Skin inoculation from bite or from contact with infected animal tissue. 1–5 days later a papule forms that ulcerates. The end result is a granulomatous reaction with regional tender lymphadenitis
  - **Oculoglandular** (least common): Self-inoculation after touching infected tissues causes painful eye swelling, exudative conjunctivitis, and lymphadenopathy
  - **Oropharyngeal/gastrointestinal:** Caused by eating, drinking, or inhaling organisms; causes membranous or exudative pharyngitis, vomiting, diarrhea, and regional lymphadenopathy
  - **Typhoidal**: Characterized by a severe flu-like illness without lymphadenopathy. No obvious site of entry identified
  - **Pneumonic** (most severe form): Abrupt onset of severe febrile illness with headache, myalgias (typically low back), sore throat, and productive cough. It progresses to pleuritic chest pain, dyspnea, and hemoptysis. CXR may initially be normal in up to 70% of patients; later findings include multilobar pneumonia, hilar lymphadenopathy, and pleural effusions with progressive granulomatous lung tissue destruction

■ Additional Studies

- Microbiology lab should be notified to grow sputum and blood cultures on cystine-rich agar
- Serology showing greater than 1:160 titers or a 4-fold increase between acute and convalascent titers

■ Differential Diagnosis
- Psittacosis, Q-fever, plague
- Because the organism is difficult to identify without proper testing, often misdiagnosed as *Haemophilus influenzae*

■ Management
- First-line: **Streptomycin or gentamicin**
- Second-line: Doxycycline, ciprofloxacin, or chloramphenicol
- Oral prophylaxis (14 days) for exposure to source: Doxycycline or ciprofloxacin
- There is no person-to-person spread
- Vaccine under investigation

■ Complications
- Rarely, granulomatous mediastinal masses
- Rhabdomyolysis, renal failure, and septic shock from liberated endotoxin

21 Prevention of Infection

Erik R. Dubberke, MD and Victoria J. Fraser, MD

Passive Immunization

Transfer of preformed antibodies into a susceptible host
- Most commonly: Transplacental transfer to developing fetus
- Prevents or treats infection or toxin-mediated disease
- Can be equine, human, or recombinant in origin
- Can be pooled immunoglobulin or disease-specific

■ Indications

Prevention of infection in patients with impaired humoral immunity: Intravenous immunoglobulin (IVIG)
- Common variable immunodeficiency, transplant recipients
- 300–500 mg/kg IVIG every 3–6 weeks IV

Botulism
Trivalent equine antitoxin (as well as supportive care)
- One vial IV + one vial intramuscularly (IM), from Centers for Disease Control (CDC)
- Human botulism immunoglobulin for infants
- Antibiotics of unproven benefit
  - May worsen infant botulism by lysing organisms in the gut

Cytomegalovirus (CMV)
CMV immunoglobulin
- Prophylaxis against reactivation in **seropositive solid-organ transplant recipients**
- Treatment of severe CMV disease in immunocompromised patients (not FDA-approved)
  - 500 mg/kg every other day for 10 doses, then twice per week for eight doses

Hepatitis A virus (HAV)
Pooled immunoglobulin
- May be less effective in areas where HAV prevalence is low
- Postexposure prophylaxis (PEP) **within 14 days of exposure**
  - Close personal contacts of patients with acute HAV
  - Ingestion of contaminated food
  - Recipient should also be vaccinated against HAV

- Nonimmune travelers visiting areas of high endemicity
- Preventable with vaccination

Hepatitis B (HBV)
Hepatitis B immunoglobulin
- PEP ideally **within 48 hours of exposure**
  - Nonimmune person after HBV surface antigen (HBsAg)-positive needle-stick injury (NSI)
  - Sexual contacts
  - Infants born to HBsAg-positive mother
- Recipient should also be **vaccinated against HBV**
- Preventable with vaccination

Parvovirus B19
Pooled immunoglobulin (IVIG)
- 400 mg/kg IV for 5 days
- Indicated for **chronic parvovirus B19** pure red cell aplasia
  - Occurs in immunocompromised patients due to AIDS, transplants, congenital, or lymphoproliferative disorders
- If recurs, maintenance therapy every 4 weeks may be needed

Rabies
Rabies immunoglobulin (RIG)
- 20 units/kg infiltrated into and around wound, rest from vial administered IM
- Postexposure to rabid animals, should also be vaccinated
- RIG-positive human diploid vaccine is 100% effective

Tetanus
Human tetanus immunoglobulin (TIG)
- 3000–6000 units IM, consider intrathecal TIG, and vaccination
- In addition to antibiotics (penicillin or metronidazole), debridement, and supportive care for disease
- After dirty, tetanus-prone wound if unknown vaccination history or fewer than 3 previous doses of vaccine, one dose of 250 units TIG IM

Vaccinia
Vaccinia immunoglobulin (VIG)
- Available through the CDC (1-770-488-7100)
- Treatment of complications of vaccinia vaccination
  - Eczema vaccinatum, ocular or severe generalized vaccinia

Varicella-Zoster Virus (VZV)
VZV immunoglobulin
- PEP: 625 units IM, administer **within 96 hours of exposure**
  - Nonimmune women exposed in first 20 weeks of pregnancy
  - Infants born to mothers who develop varicella from 5 days before through 4 days after giving birth

- Immunocompromised children without prior VZV disease or vaccination
- Non-immune adults who are immunocompromised (HIV, steroids, malignancy) or at high risk for complications
• Preventable with vaccination

West Nile Virus
• Pooled immunoglobulin from high endemicity areas (e.g., Israel)
• Human trials pending

Active Immunization

Stimulate body's host defenses to respond to an infectious agent
• Induction of humoral immunity, cell-mediated immunity, or both, achieved by administration of a vaccine
• Live, attenuated infectious agent
  - In theory, will induce an immunological response more similar to that resulting from natural infection
  - Rarely can revert back and cause disease, in general, avoid giving to immunocompromised patients and pregnant women
• Killed whole microorganisms, toxoids, or other purified extract
• Vaccine recommendation for adults depends on prior immunizations, age, potential exposures, and **comorbidities**

■ Recommended Adult Vaccinations

Hepatitis A
Inactivated HAV
• Two doses IM: At time 0 and 6 months; **85% effective**
• Should be given to nonimmune adults with the following risk factors:
  - Medical conditions: Bleeding disorders requiring clotting factor concentrates, chronic liver disease
  - Occupational: People working with HAV in research settings (consider vaccination of food handlers)
  - Behavioral: Illicit drug use (injection and noninjection), men who have sex with men
  - Other: Travel to areas of high/intermediate HAV prevalence
• Adverse reactions: Local reactions, contraindicated (CI) if known allergies to vaccine components

Hepatitis B
Purified inactivated HBsAg
• From plasma of patients with chronic hepatitis B, or
• From yeast through recombinant DNA technology
• Three doses IM: at time 0, 1, and 6 months; 75% to 90% effective
  - Decreased response associated with smoking, obesity, immunosuppression, and increasing age

- Now part of routine childhood vaccinations
- Should be given to nonimmune adults with the following risk factors:
  - Medical conditions: Hemodialysis patients, bleeding disorders requiring clotting factors, HIV, chronic liver disease
  - Occupational: **Healthcare workers** (HCWs), human tissue laboratory workers, people who work with institutionalized populations
  - Behavioral: Injection drug users, high-risk sexual activity (men who have sex with men, more than one partner in previous 6 months), all clients of sexually transmissible disease (STD) clinics
  - Other: Household contact with chronic HBV, travel to areas with high or intermediate prevalence for more than 6 months, inmates of correctional facilities
- Adverse reactions: Local reactions, no known CI

Influenza
Inactivated virus or intranasal live attenuated virus
- Use intranasal vaccine only for healthy persons aged 5–49 years (not HCWs), otherwise use inactivated virus
- Annually in the fall, **60% to 80% effective**
- Three influenza strains covered (two type A and one type B)
  - Changes depending on most common strains in community
- Indicated if ≥ 50 years old, long-term care facility residents, HCWs, pregnant women in second or third trimester during influenza season, and contacts of high-risk persons
- Indicated for all patients with chronic medical conditions (cardiac, pulmonary, renal, diabetes, hemoglobinopathy, or immunosuppression induced by medication or disease)
- Adverse reactions:
  - **Avoid in patients with severe egg allergies**
  - Intranasal live vaccine can cause mild upper respiratory infection (URI) symptoms
  - Some preparations of live attenuated vaccine associated with Bell's palsy
  - Local reactions and fever in 3–5%
  - Rare association with Guillain-Barré Syndrome

Measles, Mumps, Rubella Vaccination
Live, attenuated viruses
- Given at 12–15 months, booster at 4–6 years
- **More than 95% effective after first dose**
- Adults born before 1957 may be considered immune
  - Adults born after 1957 should receive at least one dose unless vaccinated as child, physician documented disease, or laboratory evidence of immunity

- Adults should get a second dose if:
  - Recently exposed to measles in an outbreak setting
  - Previously vaccinated with killed virus vaccine
  - Vaccinated with unknown vaccine between 1963 and 1967
  - Students in postsecondary educational institutions
  - Work in healthcare facility
  - Plan to travel internationally
- Assess immunity to rubella in women of childbearing age
- Vaccinate women with unreliable prior vaccination history
  - Advise to avoid pregnancy for 4 weeks after vaccination
  - **CI if pregnant,** although no cases of vaccine-associated neonatal rubella have been reported
- **CI in immunocompromised patients**
  - Should be administered to patients with asymptomatic or mildly symptomatic HIV
- Adverse reactions:
  - Anaphylaxis has been reported
  - More than 5% develop fevers > 103°F (39.3°C) from measles component
  - Rash in 5% from measles component
  - 25% of susceptible adult women will develop arthralgias from rubella component, 10% will develop acute arthritis
  - Rare cases of parotitis and orchitis from mumps component
  - Possible association with encephalopathy from measles component

Meningococcus
Purified capsular polysaccharide
- Serogroups A, C, Y, and W-135, 90% effective, single dose
- Consider revaccination in 3–5 years if patient at persistent risk
- Indications: Terminal complement deficiency, asplenia, travel to hyperendemic or endemic areas ("meningitis belt" of sub-Saharan Africa, Mecca, Saudi Arabia for hajj)
  - Counsel **college freshmen** and parents on risks and benefits
- Adverse reactions: Mild local reactions, no known CI

Pneumococcal Polysaccharide Vaccine
- Polysaccharide extracts of 23 most common serotypes
  - **Covers 85% to 90% of bacteremic pneumococcal isolates** in US
  - Polysaccharide vaccines induce a B cell-independent response: Booster response absent on revaccination and not effective in young children
- 60% to 80% effective
- All people ≥ 65 years old, Alaskan natives, and certain Native American populations, long-term care facility residents

- Indicated for all patients with chronic medical conditions regardless of age (cardiac, pulmonary, renal, liver, asplenia, diabetes, immunosuppression, chemotherapy with alkylating agents, antimetabolites, or long-term corticosteroids)
- One-time **booster 5 years after primary vaccination** if:
  - Chronic renal failure or nephrotic syndrome
  - Functional or anatomic asplenia
  - Immunosuppressive conditions (e.g., HIV, transplant, etc.)
  - Chemotherapy or long-term corticosteroids
  - Persons ≥ 65 years old with vaccination before the age of 65
- Adverse reactions: Local reaction in up to 50%, more severe with booster, no known CI

Polio
Live attenuated virus (OPV) or inactivated virus (IPV)

- Both more than 95% effective
- IPV only series now recommended for all children
- Due to eradication of wild-type polio in the Western Hemisphere, it is not recommended to vaccinate nonimmune adults unless they are traveling to an endemic region
  - If an adult needs vaccination, give IPV at 0, 1, and 6 months
  - Adults who are immune and traveling to an endemic region may receive an additional dose of OPV or IPV
- OPV is CI in immunocompromised, pregnant patients, and people living with immunocompromised persons
- Adverse reactions: Vaccine-associated paralytic polio rarely associated with OPV. IPV without any known significant adverse reactions

Tetanus and Diphtheria (Td)
Toxoid

- Adults with unknown history should receive series of three doses
  - First two doses are given 4 weeks apart
  - Third dose given 6–12 months after the second dose
- All adults should receive a booster every 10 years
- **Booster if last vaccination more than 5 years** prior and high-risk injury
- Adverse reactions:
  - Local reactions and fever common
  - Rarely associated with **brachial neuritis**
  - Possible association with Guillain-Barré Syndrome

Varicella
Live attenuated virus

- Two doses 4–8 weeks apart
- **86% effective against any varicella, 100% effective against severe varicella**

- Indications for adults without prior vaccination or disease:
  - Employment or residing in institutions where transmission is likely to occur (healthcare facility, daycare, preschool and elementary school, college, correctional facilities)
  - Household contact of children or immunocompromised
  - Women of child-bearing age
  - Avoid if pregnant or planning pregnancy in next 4 weeks
  - International travel
- CI in immunocompromised patients
- Adverse reactions:
  - Anaphylaxis
  - Localized or generalized varicella-like rash in 1% to 6%
  - Transmission of vaccine virus has been documented
  - Although associated with a lower risk of zoster, the varicella vaccine virus has been rarely associated with zoster

■ Vaccines with Specific Indications

See Chapter 19 for typhoid, yellow fever, Japanese encephalitis, rabies, and cholera.

Anthrax (see also Chapter 20)
- Purified protective antigen derived from avirulent nonencapsulated *B. anthracis* available in the US
- Dose at 0, 1, 6, 12, and 18 months, boosters given annually
- 92% effective against cutaneous anthrax
- Adverse reactions: Mild local reaction in 30%, severe local reaction in less than 4%, systemic reactions in 0.2%

Bacille Calmette-Guérin Vaccine (BCG)
- **Live BCG, an attenuated strain of *M. bovis,*** single dose
- Controversy regarding efficacy
  - May prevent complications of disseminated TB in children
- Not recommended in US because risk for TB infection is low, and it results in conversion of the tuberculin skin test
- CI in immunocompromised patients
- Adverse reactions: **Regional adenitis, disseminated BCG infections,** osteitis

Haemophilus influenzae type B vaccine (HIB)
- Capsular polysaccharide covalently linked to a protein carrier
- Consider in adults with functional or anatomic asplenia

Plague
Suspension of killed *Yersinia pestis* (see also Chapter 20)
- Dose at 0, 1, and 6 months, unknown efficacy
- Booster every 6 months for 1–2 years after series, then yearly

- Only persons at high risk of exposure: Laboratory workers who work with *Y. pestis*, people who work with wild animals in plague zootic areas (New Mexico, Arizona)
- CI include known hypersensitivity or previous severe reaction
- Adverse reactions: Mild local reactions common, mild systemic complaints in 20% (headache)

Smallpox
Live unattenuated vaccinia virus, 95% effective
- Single dose: Bifurcated needle with a drop of vaccine is pressed into the upper arm 15 times
- Recommended if high risk for contact with orthopoxviruses that can infect humans (smallpox, vaccinia, monkeypox, etc.)
    - Laboratory workers who work with these viruses
    - HCWs who administer and come in contact with vaccinia vaccinations
    - Voluntary for "emergency first-responders"
- Many CI: Known allergy to vaccine, eczema, heart disease, immunocompromised, pregnancy, infants less than 1 year old, moderate or severe underlying illness
- Adverse reactions:
    - Mild: Local reactions, fever, lymphadenopathy, interfering with daily activity in 30%
    - Severe: Localized vaccinia, autoinoculation, generalized vaccinia, erythema multiforme, myopericarditis
    - Life-threatening: Eczema vaccinatum, vaccinia necrosum, postvaccinal encephalitis

Chemoprophylaxis

Use of antimicrobials to prevent infection
- Postexposure or during outbreak of specific pathogen
- Related to surgical procedure
- Endocarditis prophylaxis
- Immunocompromised/special hosts

■ Postexposure Prophylaxis
Influenza
- Vaccination is recommended form of prophylaxis; chemoprophylaxis reserved for those with CI to vaccination
- Chemoprophylaxis for susceptible populations during outbreaks in addition to vaccination to protect while vaccine-induced antibodies develop (see indications for vaccination above)
- Chemoprophylaxis effective after known exposure, give for duration of outbreak or 7 days after exposure

- **Oseltamivir** 75 mg orally (PO) once a day (protects against A and B)
- Rimantadine or amantadine 100 mg PO twice daily, or daily if over 65 years old (protects against influenza A only)

Meningitis (Neisseria meningitidis and H. influenzae)

- Prophylaxis to household contacts, daycare contacts, close (1 m or less) exposure to case patient for total 4 hours or more, or exposure to case patient during procedure likely to cause aerosolization of airway secretions (e.g., intubation) without face mask
- *N. meningitidis*: Prophylaxis should be administered **within 3 days** after exposure unless previously vaccinated
  - **Rifampin** 600 mg PO twice a day for 4 days, or ciprofloxacin 500 mg PO one dose (avoid if pregnant), or ceftriaxone 250 mg IM one dose
- *H. influenzae*: Prophylaxis should be administered within 3 days after exposure unless previously vaccinated
  - Rifampin 20 mg/kg PO once a day for 4 days
  - Avoid rifampin in women on oral contraceptives; increase in hepatic metabolism of hormones can cause contraceptive failure

Hepatitis B and HIV

- See Needle-Stick Injury, below

Lyme Disease

- Consider chemoprophylaxis if partially engorged tick found on patient while in area where Lyme disease is endemic
  - Decreased erythema migrans from 3% to 0.4%
  - **Doxycycline** 200 mg PO one dose with food

Rheumatic Fever (RF)

- **Secondary prophylaxis** after episode of acute RF
  - **Benzathine penicillin G** 1.2 million units IM every 3–4 weeks, or **penicillin V** 250 mg PO twice daily, or sulfadiazine 1 g PO daily, or **erythromycin** 250 mg PO twice daily
- Duration of prophylaxis varies with manifestation of acute RF
  - If there is carditis, continue for 10 years or until 25 years old
  - If no carditis, continue for 5 years or until 18 years old

High-Risk Sexual Exposure

- Exam and baseline testing for gonorrhea, chlamydia, syphilis, HIV, HBV, *Trichomonas*; offer emergency contraception
- Ceftriaxone 125 mg IM one dose + metronidazole 2 g PO one dose + azithromycin 1 g PO one dose (or doxycycline 100 mg PO twice daily for 7 d)

- Consider HIV and HBV prophylaxis (see Needle-Stick Injury, below)
- Repeat testing for sexually transmitted diseases in 1–2 weeks. Repeat syphilis and HIV serologies at 6, 12, and 24 weeks

Varicella-Zoster Virus
- Over 50% of varicella-related deaths occur in adults
- Vaccinate adults at risk (see above)
- Administer PEP to nonimmune adults at high risk for complications and immunocompromised adults (HIV, malignancies, pregnancy, steroids)
    - VZV immunoglobulin (see above), and initiate acyclovir 800 mg PO five times daily immediately if a rash develops

■ Surgical Prophylaxis
- Prevent surgical site infections
    - Patient risk factors: Immune status, **nutritional status**, diabetes
    - High infection risk surgery: Crosses mucosal barrier
    - Significant morbidity associated with infection: Prosthetic device insertion
- Antibiotic(s) directed against flora found at surgical incision site
- Antibiotic infusion should be completed **before** first incision
    - Re-dose rapidly cleared antibiotics every 3 hours
    - Should be **discontinued within 24 hours** after the surgery
- If the patient has a beta-lactam allergy, vancomycin or clindamycin can be used when gram-positive coverage is needed, and gentamicin can be used when gram-negative coverage is needed

Cardiovascular Surgery
- Any surgery with **foreign body or prosthetic device** placement
- Cardiac surgery; prophylaxis not indicated for cardiac catheterization
- Surgeries that involve a leg groin incision
- Lower extremity amputation for ischemia
- Antibiotic: Cefazolin 1–2 g IV, or cefuroxime 1.5 g IV
    - Add vancomycin 1 g IV if high rate of methicillin-resistant *Staphylococcus aureus* (MRSA) infection

Gastrointestinal Tract Surgery
- High-risk gastroduodenal surgery (obesity, obstruction, acid suppression, abnormal motility) or high-risk biliary surgery (>70 years old, acute cholecystitis, nonfunctioning gallbladder, obstructive jaundice, common biliary duct stones)
    - Cefazolin, cefoxitin, cefotetan, or cefuroxime 1.5 g IV
    - If cholangitis, treat as infection (beta-lactam with beta-lactamase inhibitor)

Head and Neck (prophylaxis only if surgery crosses mucosa)
- Cefazolin 2 g IV, or clindamycin 600–900 mg IV + gentamicin 1.5 mg/kg IV

Obstetric/Gynecologic
- Vaginal or abdominal hysterectomy: Cefazolin, cefoxitin, cefotetan, or cefuroxime 1–2 g IV

Orthopedic
- **Antibiotic beads or cement** of **unproven** benefit
- Hip arthroplasty, spinal fusion, joint replacement
  - Cefazolin 1–2 g IV
  - Add vancomycin 1 g IV if high rate of MRSA infection

■ Endocarditis Prophylaxis

- Endocarditis prophylaxis recommendations are based on the patient's risk of developing endocarditis after a procedure associated with bacteremia
- Risk associated with:
  - Underlying cardiac abnormality
  - Likelihood of bacteremia during procedure
- Prophylaxis focuses on organisms more likely to be associated with endocarditis: Viridans streptococci, *Enterococcus* spp
- Underlying risk split into high, intermediate, and low (Table 21-1)

■ TABLE 21-1 Endocarditis Prophylaxis Based on Underlying Cardiac Abnormalities

High Risk	Intermediate Risk	Low Risk
Prophylaxis		No Prophylaxis
Prosthetic valve	MVP with regurgitation	MVP without regurgitation
Prior endocarditis	Tricuspid valve disease	
Cyanotic congenital heart disease	Pulmonary stenosis	Isolated atrial septal defect
Aortic regurgitation and stenosis (including bicuspid valves)	Asymmetric septal hypertrophy	Atherosclerotic plaques
	Age-related degenerative valve disease	CAD
Mitral regurgitation and stenosis		Previous coronary bypass grafting
PDA		Cardiac pacemaker or defibrillator
Ventricular septal defect		
Aortic coarctation		

Abbreviations: CAD, coronary artery disease; MVP, mitral valve prolapse; PDA, patent ductus arteriosus

- Procedures for which prophylaxis should be considered for high- and intermediate-risk cardiac abnormalities:
  - Dental: Extractions, gingival surgery, root canal, implant placement, cleaning if bleeding is anticipated
  - Respiratory: Tonsillectomy, surgery on respiratory mucosa, rigid bronchoscopy
  - Gastrointestinal: Sclerotherapy of varices, esophageal dilation, endoscopic retrograde cholangiopancreatography (ERCP) with obstruction present, biliary tract surgery
  - Other: Surgical procedure involving infected tissue
- Procedures for which **prophylaxis is not routinely recommended:**
  - Dental: Filling cavities, injection of local anesthetic
  - Respiratory: Intubations, flexible bronchoscopy
  - Gastrointestinal: Endoscopy, transesophageal echocardiogram
  - Genitourinary: Any procedure in absence of infection
  - Other: Cardiac catheterization, angioplasty, coronary stent placement, pacemaker/defibrillator placement, skin biopsy
- Prophylaxis for dental, respiratory, or esophageal procedures:
  - Amoxicillin 2 g PO 1 hour before procedure, or
  - Ampicillin 2 g IV 30 minutes before procedure
  - Beta-lactam allergy: Clindamycin (600 mg PO), or azithromycin (500 mg), or clarithromycin (500 mg) PO or IV 1 hour before procedure
- Prophylaxis for gastrointestinal/genitourinary procedures:
  - High-risk abnormality: Ampicillin 2 g + gentamicin 1.5 mg/kg IV 30 minutes before procedure + ampicillin 1 g IV, or amoxicillin 1 g PO 6 hours after the procedure
  - High-risk abnormality and beta-lactam allergic: Vancomycin 1 g IV and gentamicin 1.5 mg/kg IV before procedure
  - Intermediate-risk abnormality: Amoxicillin 2 g PO 1 hour before procedure, or ampicillin 2 g IV 30 minutes before procedure
  - Intermediate-risk abnormality and beta-lactam allergic: Vancomycin 1 g IV before procedure
  - Immunocompromised/special hosts: See Chapters 16 and 17 for prophylaxis in HIV, neutropenia, and transplant patients
  - Functional or anatomical asplenia: In addition to vaccination (see above), penicillin V 250 mg PO twice daily

Needle-Stick Injury

- To decrease risk of NSI
  - Avoid recapping/disassembly sharps: **Reduces risk up to 40%**
  - Double glove for procedures
  - Announce sharps passage and use a neutral zone for passage

- Know what to do if you have a NSI or body substance exposure
  - Stop what you are doing, remove gloves and check for blood
  - Wash area thoroughly with soap and water
  - Follow local procedure on how to report NSI
  - Determine need for PEP
  - Source patient high-risk characteristics include infected with known blood-borne pathogen, victim of violence, intravenous drug user, men who have sex with men, multiple heterosexual contacts, transfusion before 1985 (HIV) or 1990 (HCV), high-prevalence area
- **All source patients should be tested for HBV, HCV, and HIV**

■ HBV (preventable with vaccination)

- Risk of transmission
  - Source patient HBsAg positive, HBeAg positive: 20% to 40%
  - Source patient HBsAg positive, HBeAg negative: 1% to 6%
- Test HCW for HBsAb
- If HCW is known to have HBsAb titer 10 mIU/mL or higher at any time in the past, no further treatment is necessary
- Nonvaccinated HCW or vaccinated nonresponder HCW:
  - HBV vaccination series and one dose of HBV immunoglobulin
- Follow HBV serology at 3 and 6 months

■ HCV (PEP not available for HCV)

- Risk of transmission
  - Source patient HCV antibody-positive: 1% to 6%
  - HCV RNA positive: 10.3%
- Check HCW **HCV antibodies at baseline, 6 months, and 12 months**
- Check **HCV RNA and liver enzymes 4–6 weeks after exposure**
  - If HCW develops acute HCV, refer HCW to HCV expert for counseling and evaluation for treatment options

■ HIV (see Chapter 16)

Infection Control

■ Hand Hygiene

- Hand hygiene can be practiced through hand washing or use of alcohol-based hand hygiene products
- **Proper hand washing technique**
  - Turn on faucet, wet hands, lather soap for 15 seconds, then rinse
  - Dry hands on paper towel, turn off faucet with used towel

- Unless hands are visibly soiled, **alcohol-based hand hygiene products** can be used instead of hand washing
  - Rapidly kills vegetative bacteria
  - Alcohol-based products do not kill bacterial spores
- Hand washing should be performed after contact with a *Clostridium difficile*-positive patient
- HCW compliance with hand washing is typically less than 50%
- Proper hand hygiene before and after all patient contact; after contact with bodily fluids, mucous membranes, or nonintact skin; after removing gloves; after contact with contaminated equipment; after using the restroom and eating; and before eating, drinking, smoking, or handling food

■ Standard Precautions

- Applies to all patients
- Gloves should be worn before contact with blood, bodily fluids (except sweat), mucous membranes, and nonintact skin
- For any procedure that can generate splashes or sprays, a mask, eye protection, and a gown should be worn

■ Respiratory Hygiene/Cough Etiquette

- Prevent transmission of respiratory infections at point of first contact (triage areas, outpatient clinics, physician offices)
- Any source with respiratory symptoms
- Source patient should cough or sneeze into tissue or wear surgical mask when tolerated
- Hand hygiene after contact with respiratory secretions
- Source remains more than 3 feet away from other people if possible

■ Contact Precautions (follow standard precautions)

- Gowns and gloves worn for all contact with patient and patient's environment (masks and eye protection as indicated)
  - HCW and visitors
- Patients should be placed in isolation or cohorted with other patients with the same pathogen
- Prevent transmission of epidemiologically important organisms from an infected or colonized patient (proven or suspected)
  - Known infection or colonization with drug-resistant organism: MRSA, vancomycin-resistant enterococci, multidrug resistant gram-negative rods
  - Infectious diarrhea: *C. difficile*, *E. coli*, *Salmonella*, viral, etc.
  - Other: Group A streptococcus, lice, scabies, etc.

■ **Droplet Precautions** (follow standard precautions)
- Prevent transmission of large-particle aerosols
  - Produced when patient talks, coughs, sneezes, and during procedures (e.g., intubation), generally do not travel more than 3 feet
- Patients should be placed in isolation or cohorted
- Special air handling not required (door to room can be open)
- HCW should wear a surgical mask if within 3 feet of the patient
- Patient should wear a surgical mask before leaving the room
- **Organisms transmitted by large droplets** include: *H. influenzae, N. meningitis, Bordetella pertussis*, influenza, respiratory syncytial virus (RSV), parvovirus B19, rubella, mumps, adenovirus, group A streptococcus (pharyngitis or pneumonia), use precautions if any are known or suspected

■ **Airborne Infection Isolation Precautions** (follow standard precautions)
- Prevent transmission of droplet nuclei (5 μm or smaller)
  - Can remain suspended in air and travel prolonged distances
- Isolate patients in negative pressure room (six exchanges or more per hour)
- HCW should wear a respirator that filters 1 μm particles with an efficiency of at least 95% (N95 respirator)
- Minimize patient transportation, patient should wear a surgical mask before leaving the room
- **Organisms transmitted by droplet nuclei** include: TB, measles, smallpox, and VZV (varicella- or disseminated zoster); use precautions if any are known or suspected
  - HCW who are not immune to vaccine-preventable airborne diseases should not enter patient's room, even with personal protection

■ **Protective Environment** (follow standard precautions)
- Reduces allogeneic hematopoietic stem cell transplant recipient exposure to fungal spores: HEPA filtration of incoming air; directed room air flow; well-sealed rooms; positive pressure in patient room relative to corridor; ventilation providing 12 or more air exchanges per hour; strategies to lower dust; regular cleaning of crevices and shower heads; prohibiting flowers and plants
- Patient should wear N95 respirator if leaving protective environment

Opportunities in Internal Medicine and Adult Infectious Diseases

■ Internal Medicine Residency Training

According to the American College of Physicians (ACP) Internal Medicine Residency Database, there are currently 329 accredited categorical internal medicine residency training programs in the United States. At the completion of a 3-year residency, candidates may take the Internal Medicine Certifying Examination to become "board certified" in internal medicine.

■ Subspecialty Training

Choosing a medicine subspecialty such as infectious diseases (ID) is an important decision that has become more complex. Medicine is evolving rapidly and giving rise to an increasing number of subspecialties. Currently, 24 approved medical specialty boards grant certification in more than 120 specialized areas. Possible medicine fellowship choices include the following:

- Allergy and immunology
- Cardiology
- Interventional cardiology
- Endocrinology
- Gastroenterology
- Hematology
- Infectious diseases
- Medical oncology
- Nephrology
- Pulmonology
- Rheumatology
- Sports medicine

The duration of additional training in the standard fellowship pathway is 2–3 years (see below). This training is generally divided into 1 year of clinical training followed by 1–2 years of scholarly activity, which includes clinical or laboratory research. Some fellows augment their clinical research training with a master's degree in public health, biostatistics, or clinical epidemiology. An alternative pathway includes 2 years of general internal medicine residency training ("fast-tracking") followed by subspecialty training.

■ Adult Infectious Disease Subspecialty Training

Subspecialty training in adult ID requires 2 years of accredited fellowship training following residency, with at least 12 months of clinical training. Fellowship training in adult ID is sometimes divided into three tracks, depending on the goals of the participant and program: (1) clinician, (2) clinical investigator, and (3) basic investigator. Although only 24 months are required for certification, most clinical investigator and basic investigator track programs are about 36 months. In addition to the year of clinical activity, training requirements include research experience, exposure to a didactic curriculum, and exposure to clinical microbiology and immunology.

■ Combined Adult and Pediatric Infectious Disease Training

The American Board of Internal Medicine (ABIM) and the American Board of Pediatrics (ABP) have agreed that graduates of combined training programs in internal medicine and general pediatrics may complete ID training for each board in 1 year less than would be required of full training in both subspecialties.

■ Career Opportunities in Infectious Diseases

ID specialists may see patients in the inpatient or outpatient setting, teach medical students and residents, conduct research, or perform a combination of these activities. According to the Infectious Diseases Society of America (IDSA), the career opportunities in infectious diseases fall into four major categories: (1) **academic medicine,** with a mixture of research, teaching, administration, and clinical practice; (2) **private practice,** focusing primarily on patient care, often practicing both ID and general internal medicine; (3) **industry,** working with pharmaceutical companies to develop or improve vaccines and antimicrobial, antiviral, and antifungal agents; and (4) **public health,** working with public health agencies, including the National Institutes of Health (NIH), the Centers for Disease Control (CDC), state or local health departments, or international programs. They may investigate disease outbreaks, conduct research, educate the public, and provide leadership in the field of ID epidemiology. It is estimated that roughly half (51%) of ID physicians are employed in nonacademic clinical practices and one-third (33%) hold academic positions.

Additional information can be obtained from the ABIM (http://www.abim.org), the IDSA (http://www.idsociety.org), and the ACP (http://www.acponline.org/residency).

Review Questions and Answers

QUESTIONS

1. A 34-year-old man with no past medical history presents to the emergency department with fever for 5 days and a new rash on his chest. On exam, multiple vesicles are noted on his chest and back from below the breast to the umbilicus; there are no pustules or crusted ulcers. Which of the following is an appropriate next step in his diagnosis and management?

   A. Sending serum antibodies for herpes simplex virus (HSV)
   B. Sending serum antibodies for varicella
   C. Unroofing a vesicle, scraping the base of the lesion with a Dacron swab, and sending the specimen for viral culture and direct fluorescent antibody (DFA)
   D. Assessing HIV antibody status
   E. Initiating therapy with cidofovir

2. A 64-year-old woman presents to clinic with fever, rhinorrhea, and cough. She also notes that she has had diarrhea since returning from a Fourth of July cruise from New York to Bermuda 5 days ago. On exam, she appears ill and has marked conjunctivitis. Which of the following viral infections could be responsible for this woman's illness?

   A. Influenza A
   B. Respiratory syncytial virus (RSV)
   C. Enterovirus
   D. Norovirus
   E. Adenovirus

3. A 29-year-old woman develops fatigue, fever, and myalgias in January. Immunofluorescence of a nasal aspirate reveals influenza B. What antiviral therapy would be most appropriate?

   A. Acyclovir
   B. Cidofovir
   C. Amantadine
   D. Oseltamivir
   E. Trifluridine

4. A 19-year-old man on a hunting trip was exposed to a gunshot at close range. He was hit in the left eye with a piece of buckshot. He presents to the emergency department 4 days later with complaints

of decreased vision and worsening eye pain. On exam, he has photophobia of the left eye with significant conjunctival infection. You suspect infectious endophthalmitis following penetrating eye trauma. After calling an emergent ophthalmology consult, what is the most appropriate study to obtain?

A. Conjunctival culture
B. Skull x-ray
C. Orbital CT
D. Urine toxicologic drug screen
E. Corneal scraping for Giemsa staining

5. A 35-year-old man from Louisiana without history of unprotected sexual activity or blood transfusion presents to the emergency department in July with 72 hours of headache, neck stiffness, fever, and chills. The patient is found to have a temperature of 102.2°F (39°C). A lumbar puncture is performed and the cerebrospinal fluid (CSF) demonstrates 300 leukocytes/mm^3 with a cell count differential of 90% lymphocytes, glucose of 54 mg/dL, and protein of 60 mg/dL. The Gram stain of the CSF and bacterial culture are negative. What is the most likely cause of this patient's findings?

A. HIV
B. *Mycobacterium tuberculosis*
C. *Neisseria meningitidis*
D. Enterovirus
E. *Cryptococcus neoformans*

6. A 16-year-old girl on the high school swim team presents with a 3-day history of a draining, itchy, and slightly painful left ear. She is afebrile. Upon examination you are unable to visualize her tympanic membrane secondary to an edematous external auditory canal and squamous debris in the canal. What is the most appropriate management?

A. Admit for IV antibiotics and order a head CT scan to evaluate for mastoiditis
B. Oral amoxicillin
C. Antibiotic ear drops
D. Antibiotic and steroid ear drops
E. Urgent otolaryngology consultation

7. A 24-year-old male college student presents with a 5-day history of sore throat that has localized to his left side over the past 36 hours. He has been unable to eat or drink anything for the past 12 hours secondary to significant odynophagia. He denies dyspnea. On examination he is febrile to 101.5°F (38.6°C), has left anterior tonsillar and palate fullness with erythema, and a palpable lymph node. What is the most appropriate initial management?

A. Rapid strep test followed by otolaryngology surgical consultation
B. Neck CT scan with IV contrast
C. Oral amoxicillin or azithromycin and discharge home with close follow-up

D. Urgent intubation for airway protection

E. Medical admission for IV antibiotics and hydration

8. A 55-year-old man remains hospitalized for parenteral nutrition via a percutaneously inserted central venous catheter following hemicolectomy for colon cancer. He develops fever. On exam, he has a new murmur. A "HACEK" organism is isolated from culture, raising your suspicion for endocarditis. Which of the following bacteria is considered a HACEK organism?

A. *Acinetobacter lwoffi*

B. *Citrobacter koseri*

C. *Haemophilus influenzae* type b

D. *Kakabacter* spp

E. *Eikenella corrodens*

9. A 78-year-old nursing home resident with a history of coronary artery disease, dementia, and chronic renal insufficiency is admitted to the hospital with fever, right-sided costovertebral angle tenderness, delirium, and a urinalysis consistent with infection. Which of the following would not be an appropriate component of her hospital care?

A. Treatment with an IV quinolone antibiotic

B. Removal of an indwelling Foley catheter and utilization of intermittent straight catheterizations for bladder retention

C. Spiral CT scan in the emergency department to rule out kidney stones

D. Renal ultrasound only if there is a delay in clinical improvement

E. Urine Gram stain and culture

10. A homeless 45-year-old alcoholic comes to the emergency department complaining of uncomfortable skin lesions on his face and arms that have been present for about 5 days. He is unkempt and had numerous erythematous lesions with vesicles, pustules, and honey-colored crusts on his face and arms. Methicillin-resistant *Staphylococcus aureus* (MRSA) is prevalent in the community. Which of the following would be the most appropriate treatment?

A. Topical mupirocin

B. Oral amoxicillin-clavulanate

C. Oral trimethoprim-sulfamethoxazole (TMP/SMX)

D. Oral cephalexin

E. Oral vancomycin

11. A 34-year-old male and his 28-year-old wife come into your office complaining of itchy red bumps present on the trunk and extremities. They have a hot tub at home, which they used 2 days before. On examination they have papules and pustules around the hair follicles on the trunk and limbs. The face, neck, palms, soles, and mucous membranes are unaffected. The most likely organism present in the skin lesions and the hot tub water is:

A. *Malassezia furfur*

B. *Streptococcus pyogenes*

C. *Pseudomonas aeruginosa*
D. *Escherichia coli*
E. *Candida albicans*

12. A 62-year-old homeless man with longstanding, poorly controlled diabetes, peripheral vascular disease, and renal insufficiency is admitted with fever, chills, elevated WBC count, and a draining foot ulcer. The ulcerative lesion on the left great toe drains purulent, foul-smelling material, and is associated with erythema and necrotic tissue. MRI reveals cortical destruction, periosteal reaction, and surrounding soft tissue changes. A diagnosis of acute osteomyelitis is made. Which of the following is the most appropriate therapeutic intervention?

    A. Vancomycin
    B. Ceftazidime
    C. Ticarcillin-clavulanate
    D. Amputate the foot
    E. Penicillin

13. A 53-year-old man, hospitalized for appendicitis, is receiving parenteral nutrition via a central venous catheter. He develops fever and chills. Central venous catheter and peripheral blood cultures reveal *S. aureus* growing 10 hours and 15 hours, respectively, after the blood culture was obtained. What is the most likely source of the bloodstream infection?

    A. Pneumonia
    B. Urinary tract infection (UTI)
    C. Intra-abdominal abscess
    D. Central venous catheter
    E. Periodontal abscess

14. A 64-year-old man with stage IV non-Hodgkin's lymphoma spikes a fever to 100.4°F (38°C) 7 days after chemotherapy (CHOP regimen: cyclophosphamide, doxorubicin, vincristine, and prednisone) is started. His only complaint is chills. You carefully examine him and note tachycardia, however the rest of the exam is essentially normal. His WBC count earlier in the day was 400/mm^3. Which of the following antimicrobial is most appropriate as empiric therapy for this patient?

    A. Vancomycin
    B. Ceftriaxone
    C. Ampicillin-sulbactam
    D. Azithromycin
    E. Cefepime

15. A 29-year-old woman who is 20 weeks pregnant is here for a routine obstetric follow-up. She has been feeling well and physical examination is unremarkable. Screening urine culture grew >10^5 cfu/mL of *E. coli*. What is the most appropriate management?

    A. Treat with oral levofloxacin
    B. Obtain ultrasound study of urinary tract

    C. Treat with oral amoxicillin

    D. Take no action as she is asymptomatic

    E. Advise her to drink cranberry juice

16. Which of the following is a correct match concerning tick-borne illnesses?

    A. Lyme disease–Most common in the fall season (i.e., September through November)

    B. Ehrlichiosis–Classic triad of fever, headache, and rash

    C. Colorado tick fever–Majority have a rash

    D. Babesiosis–Infection of WBCs

    E. Rocky Mountain spotted fever–Obligate intracellular bacteria

17. A healthy 27-year-old woman, G1 P0 and 22 weeks into a normal gestation, is admitted to the hospital for fever, malaise, and diarrhea. She was born and raised in rural Ghana, then moved to the US for graduate school 3 years ago. She just visited her home village for the first time, and 1 day after returning she developed once- or twice-daily rigors, sweats, chills, and watery diarrhea; acetaminophen has not helped. Watery brown diarrhea followed. She has no significant past medical history or allergies, and takes only prenatal vitamins. A thin blood smear shows red blood cells (RBCs) of normal size containing small ring forms; some RBCs contain more than one ring each. Which of the following is true regarding this patient?

    A. The teratogenic toxicity of antimalarial drugs precludes their use in this patient

    B. This single slide is not specific, and PCR-based assays are required to confirm the diagnosis

    C. Fetal demise is highly likely without prompt treatment

    D. The species of *Plasmodium* cannot be ascertained from this film; molecular typing is required to rule out falciparum malaria

    E. Neither her chaotic fever nor her diarrhea is consistent with *Plasmodium* infection, and another diagnosis should be sought

18. A 54-year-old man presents as a new patient at an urgent care clinic asking for vaccinations in anticipation of a vacation in Latin America in 2 weeks. His medical problems include hypertension, obesity, and insulin-requiring diabetes mellitus. He was vaccinated against meningitis 10 years ago, before traveling to Saudi Arabia, and he wonders if he needs a booster immunization. Which of the following is the most appropriate advice to offer this patient?

    A. Because of the high incidence of traveler's diarrhea in this region, prophylactic fluoroquinolone antibiotics should be prescribed for the duration of the trip

    B. Due to recent federal transportation security regulations, insulin syringes cannot be carried onto flights originating in or departing from the US

    C. Because it has been more than 5 years since his first meningitis injection, a booster should be included in his regimen now

D. Although he has diabetes, yellow fever vaccination should be offered

E. Discussing sexual practices is inappropriate with this asymptomatic new patient

19. A 47-year-old man from Arizona who works in international business presents for evaluation of multiple skin lesions. Physical exam reveals multiple maculopapular lesions on the face and extremities, all in the same stage of development. Oropharyngeal inspection reveals multiple resolving ulcerative lesions. The patient states that several days prior he came down with a high fever, diffuse myalgias, and headaches that have resolved. What is the most appropriate management?

A. Reassure the patient he has varicella

B. Place in respiratory isolation and begin treatment for pneumonic plague

C. Recommend conservative therapy for a flu-like viral illness and explain the rash is a nonspecific viral exanthem

D. Obtain as many samples of the lesions as possible to send to the lab for analysis

E. Place in negative-pressure isolation room with contact and respiratory precautions and contact the hospital and local infection control directors

20. A 38-year-old male presents for evaluation of painful nodules in his left axilla and an ulcerative lesion on the dorsum of his left hand. These events occurred following a weeklong hunting trip to Colorado. Examination shows a tender, 3-cm indurated shallow ulcer with granulomatous edges on the hand, and multiple 1–2-cm lymph nodes in the left axilla. Which one of the following presumptive diagnosis/empiric treatment pairings is reasonable to consider while completing definitive testing?

A. Variola major, treat with IV cidofovir

B. Bubonic plague, treat with PO oseltamivir

C. Cutaneous anthrax, treat with IV azithromycin

D. Cellulitis, treat with IV rifampin

E. Tularemia, treat with IV gentamicin

21. In the early fall, a 27-year-old woman presents with high fevers, malaise, productive cough, and hemoptysis. Within 24 hours of admission, her clinical course rapidly deteriorates, progressing to respiratory failure and sepsis. Which of the following agents is most likely

A. Human metapneumovirus

B. BK virus

C. Plague

D. Smallpox

22. Which one of the following is true regarding adult vaccinations?

A. Patients with HIV should not receive pneumococcal polysaccharide vaccine boosters because of their immunocompromised state

B. Adults should receive a second dose of the measles, mumps, and rubella (MMR) vaccination if they were previously vaccinated with a killed virus vaccine

C. The influenza inactivated virus vaccine is indicated for all pregnant women during the influenza season

D. Healthcare workers should receive hepatitis A vaccinations given their likelihood of encountering this disease among their patients

E. Adults with a high-risk injury do not require a tetanus and diphtheria (Td) toxoid vaccination booster as long as the last vaccination was within the last 10 years

23. A patient with HIV is found to have a CD4+ cell count of 95 cells/μL and a viral load of 400,000 copies/μL. The decision is made to start highly active antiretroviral therapy (HAART), with two nucleoside reverse transcriptase inhibitors (NRTI), as well as a protease inhibitor. Which of the following NRTI combinations would be a good choice?

A. AZT and 3TC
B. AZT and D4T
C. 3TC and FTC
D. D4T and DDI
E. Spare the protease inhibitor and begin a triple NRTI regimen

24. A 25-year-old man with a history of injection drug use presents with a 4-day history of increasing right buttock pain. He denies fever and chills. His physical exam is notable for a 5 cm × 5 cm warm, erythematous lesion with central fluctuance on his right buttock. Incision and drainage is performed, with the Gram stain revealing gram-positive cocci in clusters. What is the most appropriate empiric antibiotic therapy in this patient while awaiting culture and susceptibility results?

A. Penicillin
B. Cephalexin
C. Amoxicillin-clavulanic acid
D. TMP/SMX
E. Levofloxacin

25. Which of the following describes the mechanism of penicillin resistance in *Streptococcus pneumoniae*?

A. Efflux of the drug out of the bacteria
B. Alteration of the penicillin binding protein (PBP) target
C. Decreased permeability of the bacteria to the drug
D. Alteration of the ribosomal target
E. Expression of a beta-lactamase that cleaves penicillin

ANSWER KEY

1. C	10. C	19. E
2. E	11. C	20. E
3. D	12. C	21. C
4. C	13. D	22. B
5. D	14. E	23. A
6. D	15. C	24. D
7. A	16. E	25. B
8. E	17. C	
9. C	18. D	

ANSWERS

1. **C. The cellular material at the base of vesicular lesions is the best specimen to send for identification. The direct fluorescent antibody test is a sensitive, specific, and rapid way to diagnose herpes zoster (which is caused by reactivation of varicella-zoster virus [VZV]).**

   The most common cause of an adult presenting with a history of fever and multidermatomal vesicular rash is herpes zoster, caused by reactivation of **VZV**. Herpes simplex virus also may present with a vesicular rash, but it is unlikely to be widely disseminated in the absence of primary infection or immunocompromise. Serum antibodies are not diagnostic for primary HSV infection, as it typically takes 21 days to develop antibodies to the virus. Direct fluorescent antibody test (answer C) can detect both varicella and herpes simplex viruses.

   By adulthood, more than 90% of people have varicella virus antibodies. Therefore, positive varicella antibody titers could not confirm the diagnosis. However, the absence of varicella antibodies in this patient (assuming that he does not have an immunocompromising condition that affects antibody production) would lower your suspicion for this diagnosis.

   As disseminated herpes zoster is unusual in immunocompetent young patients, a patient diagnosed with disseminated herpes zoster should undergo assessment of HIV risk factors and antibody status. However, this patient has localized not disseminated herpes zoster. The first step should be to confirm that the rash represents localized herpes zoster.

   The early initiation of antiviral therapy in patients with herpes zoster may decrease the risk of post-herpetic neuralgia and the duration of lesions. Although cidofovir, a competitive inhibitor of DNA polymerase, has activity against several viruses including varicella, cytomegalovirus (CMV), Epstein-Barr virus (EBV), human herpesvirus 6 (HHV-6), HHV-8, papillomavirus, poxviruses, and adenovirus, it is **never** considered first-line therapy for varicella-associated illness. Other extremely effective and dramatically less nephrotoxic agents are available, such as acyclovir, valacyclovir, or famciclovir.

2. **E. Adenoviral infection may occur year-round, as opposed to other viral causes of upper respiratory infection (URI) that are restricted to fall, winter, or spring months. The combination of URI symptoms and diarrhea is classic for adenovirus, as is the finding of conjunctivitis.**

    Influenza is restricted to the fall and winter months in the Northern Hemisphere and is an uncommon cause of conjunctivitis.

    RSV usually occurs in late fall, winter, or spring in the Northern Hemisphere and is not a typical cause of diarrhea.

    Enterovirus infections commonly occur in the summer months in the Northern Hemisphere and may cause diarrhea, but are not typically associated with upper respiratory symptoms.

    Noroviruses are commonly acquired on cruises, but do not cause upper respiratory symptoms.

3. **D. Both oseltamivir (Tamiflu) and zanamivir (Relenza) specifically target the neuraminidase protein common to influenza A and B viruses. They ultimately interfere with deaggregation and release of viral progeny. Oseltamivir is administered orally. Zanamivir is delivered to the respiratory tract by oral inhalation. When started within 36 hours of illness, these compounds reduce the duration of illness by 1–2 days. Perhaps more importantly, prophylactic administration can prevent influenza in exposed contacts.**

    Acyclovir competitively inhibits viral DNA polymerase and terminates DNA chain elongation. It is active against HSV-1 and -2, varicella, CMV, and EBV.

    Cidofovir has activity against adenovirus, CMV, EBV, HSV, varicella, and, potentially, smallpox. It is associated with significant nephrotoxicity.

    Amantadine, like rimantadine, inhibits ion channel function of the M2 protein, which blocks viral uncoating during endocytosis at low concentrations. At higher lysosomal concentrations, viral fusion is inhibited. At normal doses this agent has activity against influenza A. Although this agent has some activity against influenza B at very high in vitro concentrations, the clinical effectiveness against influenza B is quite poor.

    Trifluridine monophosphate irreversibly inhibits thymidylate synthetase, and trifluridine triphosphate inhibits viral and cellular DNA polymerases. It is most often used to treat HSV keratitis; it is active against HSV-1 and -2, CMV, vaccinia, and adenoviruses.

4. **C. Orbital CT would identify a residual foreign body. Anterior chamber or vitreous fluid should be sent for Gram stain and aerobic,**

anaerobic, and fungal cultures. This patient also requires antibiotic therapy with a combination with vancomycin and either ciprofloxacin or ceftazidime.

In a patient with endophthalmitis following penetrating ocular trauma, a conjunctival culture would not be useful. A more appropriate specimen would be an anterior chamber or vitreous fluid sample (obtained by an ophthalmologist) sent for Gram stain and culture.

Skull x-ray may reveal a radio-opaque intraocular foreign body. However, it would not provide sufficient anatomic detail, and is not the appropriate test in a patient who may have a metallic intraocular foreign body.

Urine toxicologic drug screen is an important consideration in a patient likely to require operative intervention. However, giving the sight-threatening nature of endophthalmitis in a seemingly coherent patient, this would not be an appropriate use of time.

Giemsa staining of a corneal scraping would be useful to detect multinucleated giant cells that characterize HSV infection, including keratitis. Given the history suggesting penetrating trauma, HSV infection is not likely to be the cause of this infection, making such testing unnecessary.

5. **D. Aseptic meningitis is characterized by an acute onset of meningeal symptoms. CSF examination will often demonstrate pleocytosis with lymphocytic predominance. The CSF glucose will often be normal while the CSF protein may be normal or elevated. The causes of aseptic meningitis are numerous, however, enteroviruses account for over half the cases. Enterovirus meningitis typically occurs in the summer and is self-limited.**

This patient did not have any risk factors for HIV infection and also did not present with an illness specific to immunocompromised patients. Illness that would be more likely to suggest HIV infection include cryptococcal meningitis, CMV retinitis or encephalitis, and *Pneumocystis jiroveci* pneumonia.

M. tuberculosis meningitis is characterized by profound hypoglycorrachia (low CSF glucose) and a dramatically elevated CSF protein (often over 1000 mg/dL). In an otherwise healthy patient without typical CSF findings, tuberculous meningitis would be unlikely.

N. meningitidis usually presents with signs and symptoms of severe illness. The classic purpura fulminans rash occurs in many cases. CSF findings with meningococcal meningitis are similar to other bacterial causes of meningitis; the CSF white blood cell count typically exceeds 1000/mm³ with a neutrophil predominance and the CSF glucose is usually below 40 mg/dL.

C. neoformans, a yeast-like fungus, causes chronic meningitis in immunocompromised patients. Patients with AIDS account for most cases, although an increasing number of cases are now being diagnosed in solid organ transplant recipients.

6. **D.** This patient's symptoms are consistent with acute otitis externa. This is a common condition in people who swim or wear hearing aids. The organisms responsible are usually *Pseudomonas aeruginosa*, *Staphylococcus aureus*, or other gram-negatives. The treatment of choice is an antibiotic ear drop with a steroid component (such as neomycin/polymyxin/hydrocortisone or CiproDex). The steroid will help diminish the canal edema and pruritus. In addition, dry ear precautions should be followed, and those wearing hearing aids should be encouraged to limit their use as much as possible until symptoms improve.

This patient does not have the clinical signs or symptoms of mastoiditis. This would include a 10–14 day history of ear complaints, a tender/edematous/erythematous mastoid process, and often a protuberant ear. If this were the case, an otolaryngology consult would be warranted.

Amoxicillin would be used as first line management for acute otitis media. Unless this patient had other symptoms to suggest acute otitis media (such as significant otalgia and/or fever), then oral antibiotics are not generally indicated.

Antibiotic ear drops (without steroids) would be most appropriate in cases of chronic suppurative otitis media where there is a tympanic membrane perforation without significant external auditory canal edema.

In general, otitis externa can be managed in the primary care setting. On occasion, the external auditory canal edema can cause such stenosis that the otic drops cannot penetrate into the canal. In this situation, a routine otolaryngology consult may result in suctioning of debris from the canal and placement of an otowick to allow transfer of the drop medially into the canal.

7. **A.** This patient most likely has developed a peritonsillar abscess. Classically, a peritonsillar abscess develops after 3–7 days of pharyngitis. It is very rare to develop a peritonsillar abscess prior to 48 hours of symptoms. Patients complain of unilateral throat pain and have significant trismus secondary to inflammation of the pterygoid muscles. Likely pathogens are usually *Streptococcus*. In most emergency departments, surgical consultation is required for either needle aspiration or incision and drainage of the abscess. One dose of IV antibiotics (such as clindamycin), IV hydration, and possible IV steroids are often given in the emergency department prior to procedure. If the patient can drink post-procedure, then they can be discharged home with oral antibiotics (clindamycin) for 7–10 days.

Although neck CT scans with IV contrast are used routinely to evaluate for neck abscesses, in general they are not necessary in an uncomplicated peritonsillar abscess, as it should be a clinical diagnosis.

Oral antibiotics would not yield appropriate penetration of the abscess cavity to yield a likely cure.

This patient did not complain of any dyspnea. In general, peritonsillar abscesses are drained at the bedside without intubation if the patient can be cooperative (not applicable to children, who are often drained in the operating room). The act of intubation can inadvertently open the abscess cavity while the patient is sedated and unable to adequately protect their airway from aspiration of the abscess purulence. Nonetheless, peritonsillar abscesses can eventually lead to airway compromise, and if they do, constitute an airway and surgical emergency.

Though IV antibiotics and hydration may help, in general any abscess needs to be surgically drained to yield the best chance for cure.

8. **E. The HACEK organisms are oral gram-negative bacilli that cause up to 10% of cases of native valve endocarditis. The acronym HACEK represents the following organisms:** *Haemophilus* spp (*H. parainfluenzae, H. aphrophilus,* and *H. paraphrophilus*), *Actinobacillus actinomycetemcomitans, Cardiobacterium hominis, Eikenella corrodens,* and *Kingella* spp. **These organisms have specific nutritional requirements and, as a result, grow slowly in routine culture medium. Therefore, when endocarditis is suspected, blood cultures should be retained for at least 2 weeks to allow for growth of a HACEK organism. These organisms are best treated with a third-generation cephalosporin.**

Acinetobacter spp are gram-negative rods that cause nosocomial bloodstream infections. This bacteria does not have fastidious growth requirements.

Citrobacter koseri, a gram-negative rod, causes a wide variety of infections including nosocomial bloodstream infections and urinary tract infections (UTIs). In young infants, this organism is associated with meningitis and brain abscesses.

H. influenzae type b formerly caused serious infections including meningitis, bloodstream infections, and cellulitis. Since introduction of routine *H. influenzae* type b immunization, infections due to this organism are rare.

Kakabacter? Sorry, we made this name up.

9. **C. This patient has acute pyelonephritis and requires admission for IV antibiotics. Unless there are specific signs and symptoms to suggest kidney stones (e.g., abdominal pain radiating to the groin), immediate, more sophisticated imaging studies are usually not necessary if patient responds rapidly to antibiotics.**

In this elderly patient with multiple medical problems, acute pyelonephritis should be treated with parenteral antibiotics. Quinolones are good choices given their penetration into the genitourinary system.

She has acute symptomatic pyelonephritis, and her Foley catheter should be removed during treatment of her infection. If necessary, the use of intermittent straight catheterizations is appropriate.

If the patient does not respond rapidly to antibiotics, more sophisticated imaging studies (e.g., CT scan or renal ultrasound) should be done.

Urine Gram stain and culture are often helpful in determining bacterial etiology and appropriate treatment regimens.

10. C. Oral TMP/SMX, as well as doxycycline and clindamycin, are often effective against both methicillin-sensitive and methicillin-resistant strains. The choice among these is arbitrary. Doxycycline and TMP/SMX are inexpensive, generally well tolerated, and taken twice daily, features that make therapy convenient and easily remembered. Clindamycin can cause diarrhea, but *Clostridium difficile* colitis is very uncommon in outpatients, in whom this organism is rarely part of the bowel flora.

Topical mupirocin is quite effective in superficial skin infections caused by either methicillin-sensitive or methicillin-resistant *S. aureus*. However, the presence of numerous lesions on several areas of the body makes its use inconvenient. Additionally, the high cost can be prohibitive for many patients. Topical mupirocin is often applied intranasally in patients with intranasal *S. aureus* colonization undergoing hemodialysis or cardiac surgery. This pre-preprocedure application has been shown to decrease the incidence of postoperative surgical site infections in these patient populations.

This patient has nonbullous impetigo, which is usually caused by *S. aureus*. Since methicillin-resistant strains are common in this patient's community, the drug choice should be an agent active against such strains, which oral cephalexin and amoxicillin-clavulanate are not.

Although vancomycin has excellent activity against methicillin-sensitive and methicillin-resistant *S. aureus* strains, only the intravenous form achieves therapeutic serum levels. Oral vancomycin has poor gastrointestinal tract absorption, making it ineffective in treating skin/soft tissue infections, but excellent at treating *C. difficile* diarrhea.

11. C. Achieving adequate halogen levels (e.g., chlorine), used to inhibit bacterial growth in swimming pools, hot tubs, and whirlpools is difficult because of agitation and aeration of water, elevated water temperatures, and, sometimes, large numbers of bathers. When decontamination fails, *P. aeruginosa* proliferates rapidly in the warm water. The skin lesions typically appear about 48 hours after exposure and usually do not involve the face, because most people do not submerge their heads in the water for a significant time while in the hot tub. The skin lesions, which tend to be especially numerous where the bathing suits are most snug, are self-limited and do not require antimicrobial therapy. To prevent future attacks, the hot tub requires careful maintenance, which means keeping the pH of the water between 7.2 and 7.8 and sustaining free chlorine levels over 0.5 mg/L.

M. furfur is associated with bloodstream infections in patients receiving parenteral nutrition. It is also associated with superficial infections of the skin. It is not associated with cellulitis or folliculitis.

S. pyogenes is classically associated with impetigo and cellulitis. It may also cause folliculitis, however, it is not associated with hot tub folliculitis.

E. coli and *C. albicans* are not associated with cellulitis or folliculitis in immunocompetent patients.

12. **C. Diabetic foot ulcers usually show a mixed aerobic and anaerobic infection on deep tissue culture. Thus antibiotic choice needs to reflect this particular pathology. Ticarcillin-clavulanate, piperacillin-tazobactam, and imipenem would all be considered appropriate choices. Six weeks of parenteral antibiotics are usually necessary. In some select patients with known good compliance and follow-up, a regimen of 2 weeks IV antibiotics followed by 4–6 weeks oral antibiotics may be appropriate. In diabetic patients with documented peripheral vascular disease, revascularization plays an important role in the management of diabetic foot ulcers and in avoiding the need for amputation.**

    Diabetic foot ulcers usually show mixed aerobic and anaerobic infection. Vancomycin has excellent gram-positive activity but does not cover gram-negative or anaerobic organisms. Ceftazidime has excellent gram-negative activity but does not cover either *S. aureus* or anaerobes particularly well. Penicillin has fair anaerobic activity. However, most *S. aureus* strains are penicillin resistant due to beta-lactamase production by the organism. Penicillin also does not have good activity against gram-negative organisms. The combination of all three of these drugs would be effective (but impractical and expensive).

    Patients with poor healing and revascularization and worsening, recalcitrant, or recurrent infection may ultimately require bone debridement. Amputation would be considered as a last resort.

13. **D. The differential time to positivity is defined as the difference in time it takes for a blood culture drawn through a central venous catheter and a culture drawn through a peripheral vein to become positive. The "differential time to positivity" in this case is +5 hours. Earlier growth from the central venous catheter by more than 2 hours suggests that this is a catheter-related bloodstream infection. Differential time to positivity of more than 2 hours has a sensitivity of 80% to 90% in diagnosing a catheter-related bloodstream infection. *S. aureus* is a common cause of catheter-related bloodstream infections. The appropriate management in this case includes removal of the catheter and an echocardiogram to exclude endocarditis.**

    Although other foci of infection such as pneumonia, UTI, and intra-abdominal abscesses can cause a concomitant bloodstream infection, *S. aureus* is an unusual organism in such circumstances.

More common organisms would be *S. pneumoniae* (pneumonia), *E. coli* (urinary tract or intra-abdominal infections), anaerobes (intra-abdominal or periodontal infections), or polymicrobial infections (intra-abdominal or periodontal infections).

14. **E. Fever in a neutropenic host requires prompt initiation of empiric antimicrobial therapy with activity against *P. aeruginosa*.**

    While vancomycin is sometimes added to an antipseudomonal agent when infection with gram-positive organisms is suspected, it is not appropriate to be used as a single agent.

    Ceftriaxone, a third-generation cephalosporin, is active against many gram-positive and gram-negative bacteria. However, it is inactive against *P. aeruginosa*, an important consideration in the febrile patient with chemotherapy-associated neutropenia.

    Ampicillin-sulbactam offers activity against most gram-positive bacteria, anaerobic organisms, and some gram-negative bacteria. It is not active against *P. aeruginosa*.

    Azithromycin has no activity against *Pseudomonas*. It is frequently used to treat community-acquired respiratory tract infections.

15. **C. Bacteriuria in pregnancy frequently progresses to pyelonephritis, and is associated with complications such as premature delivery and chorioamnionitis. Treatment is necessary even if the patient is asymptomatic. Amoxicillin is usually active against *E. coli* and safely administered in pregnancy.**

    Although fluoroquinolones such as levofloxacin are often used to treat UTIs in adults, its use is contraindicated during pregnancy, because it is associated with fetal cartilage toxicity.

    Imaging of urinary tract is not necessary in this patient. It may be considered in cases of recurrent UTIs to rule out anatomical abnormalities and abscesses.

    Bacteriuria in pregnancy warrants treatment regardless of symptoms.

    Cranberry juice can be effective in prevention of UTIs, however it does not treat bacteriuria.

16. **E. *Rickettsia rickettsii* and *Rickettsia parkeri* are fastidious pleomorphic gram-negative rods that are obligate intracellular bacteria.**

    Lyme disease most often occurs from May through August.

    Ehrlichiosis is considered the "spotless fever" (less than a third of patients develop rash). It typically includes high fever, malaise, myalgia, arthralgia, abdominal pain, thrombocytopenia, elevated liver function tests, and regional lymphadenopathy. Rocky Mountain spotted fever has the classic triad of fever, headache, and rash in a patient with a recent tick bite.

    Patients with Colorado tick fever have an abrupt onset of fevers, chills, headache, myalgias, and weakness. Only 15% of patients have a rash.

    The Babesiosis sporozoite enters erythrocytes. Ehrlichiosis is characterized by infection of WBCs.

17. **C. Her clinical picture, combined with exposure history, lack of medical prophylaxis, waning immunity, and pregnancy, are all highly suggestive of malaria. The thin blood smear shows RBCs of normal size, some of which contain multiple ring forms, features diagnostic of falciparum malaria. Because of the high risks involved in severe falciparum malaria in pregnancy, some form of antimalarial therapy is indicated for the health of both mother and fetus. Although no antimalarial drugs are considered "category A" for safety in gestation, many experts believe that 5 days of oral quinine and clindamycin is a safe combination in pregnancy, if drug-induced hypoglycemia is carefully avoided**

    The appearance of this thin blood smear is diagnostic of falciparum malaria: Although PCR of blood is both highly sensitive and specific for all *Plasmodium* infections, it is expensive, time-consuming, and does not quantify the burden of parasitemia.

    The appearance of this thin blood smear is diagnostic of falciparum malaria. Although sequencing can distinguish between the four species of *Plasmodium* that infect humans, we already have an answer with the smear; a molecular approach is unnecessary, expensive, time-consuming, and does not quantify the burden of parasitemia.

    Falciparum malaria is said to cause "tertian" fever (every 48 hours), but this feature is often absent during early infection; only after the first few days or week will the parasites synchronize their life cycles and cause regular fever spikes. And although the mechanism remains unclear, malaria often presents with diarrhea.

18. **D. The yellow fever vaccine contains live-attenuated virus, and carries a very small risk of neurotropic or viscerotropic disease. Vaccination is contraindicated in patients who are under 9 months old or over 70 years, allergic to eggs, pregnant, or severely immunocompromised (e.g., AIDS). If this patient has none of these conditions, and his itinerary includes areas endemic for yellow fever, he should be vaccinated.**

    Although the incidence of acute traveler's diarrhea among Americans visiting Latin America approaches 50%, most cases are benign and self-limited. A treatment course of antibiotics (e.g., levofloxacin 500 mg PO daily for 3 days) can be offered in case patients develop diarrhea associated with fever, abdominal pain, and bloody or purulent stool; however, prophylactic antibiotics are not routinely advised. (Note: prophylactic bismuth subsalicylate 2 tabs four times daily may reduce incidence of traveler's diarrhea by 60%.)

    Because insulin is a life-sustaining medication, no such regulations exist. However, in case of unforeseen medical emergencies, it is always advisable to document your patient's medical conditions, medications, and allergies in a brief letter.

    The meningitis vaccine currently available in the US provides partial immunity against *N. meningitidis* serotypes A, C, Y, and W-135.

Although documentation of this vaccination is required among pilgrims to Mecca during the hajj, the vaccine is not offered routinely among normal adults; its important role is among asplenic patients and young adults leaving home for closely cohorted living situations (e.g., college dormitories or military barracks). Protection usually does wane after several years, but boosters are not recommended.

Americans have a higher risk of acquiring sexually transmitted diseases when they travel abroad. Frank, nonjudgmental counseling about risk reduction strategies, including barrier contraceptive use, is indicated.

19. **E. For a patient presenting with diffuse maculopapular lesions, all in the same stage of healing, it is critical to consider smallpox. Treatment consists of promptly isolating the patient in a negative-pressure room under strict contact and respiratory contact precautions. The classic prodromal symptoms of fever, myalgias, and oral lesions were reported. Although the disease has not been reported in over 20 years, the current era of bioterrorism must make us reconsider the diagnosis. Contacting local public health officials will facilitate confirmatory testing and obtaining the vaccinia vaccine.**

Varicella has characteristic lesions that are different stages of healing, and usually arise centrally, on the chest and trunk, and spread distally.

Pneumonic plague is a rare but serious infection caused by *Yersinia pestis* and should be considered in this patient from the southwest US. However, skin lesions/rashes are not seen in any of the three forms of plague: bubonic, pneumonic, or septicemic. Prominent lymphadenopathy is notable with *Yersinia* infection.

Careful consideration of diffuse maculopapular lesions should now include smallpox and other poxviruses (e.g., monkeypox) before telling a patient they have a benign condition. The skin lesions seen in smallpox infection are extremely infectious.

When smallpox infection is being seriously considered as a diagnosis, collection of any skin samples should be performed under strict contact and respiratory precautions, and arrangements made for safe transport to an appropriate laboratory.

20. **E. A hunting history in the setting of an ulcerative skin lesion and notable lymphadenopathy is a typical scenario for the glandular form of tularemia. Initial treatment options include IV gentamicin or streptomycin, or doxycycline, or ciprofloxacin.**

Variola major, the typical form of smallpox, is characterized by a febrile illness that follows an asymptomatic 7–17-day incubation period. Oropharyngeal ulcerative lesions are the first cutaneous manifestation of exposure, with the characteristic maculopapular rash appearing 2–3 days later. The vesicular and subsequent pustular lesions follow 3–8 days later, all in the same stage of development. Treatment for smallpox is supportive, with strict isolation precautions warranted, as well as prompt vaccinia vaccination for the patient and all proximal contacts the patient has had in the past 3–4 weeks. Cidofovir is an investigational drug, not approved for use in suspected smallpox cases.

Bubonic plague does present with notable lymphadenopathy (buboes), and a history of direct exposure to animals that could be infected with fleas, makes consideration of bubonic plague reasonable. Treatment options include IV gentamicin or streptomycin, or oral doxycycline or a fluoroquinolone. Oseltamivir is an antiviral agent often used to treat infections caused by influenza.

Cutaneous anthrax is not uncommon in occupational and recreational activities involving direct contact with animals that are likely to have flea infestations. The skin lesion results from spore inoculation, requiring direct contact with the source, followed by toxin production and ultimately vesicle formation that coalesces to an ulcerative lesion that develops an eschar. Initial treatment consists of IV doxycycline or ciprofloxacin—not azithromycin.

Cellulitis is commonly treated with antibiotics, such as ampicillin-sulbactam, that provide coverage for gram-positive skin flora such as *Streptococcus* and *Staphylococcus* while additional testing is pursued. Although rifampin has good gram-positive activity, it is never used as monotherapy to treat cellulitis because of the rapid development of resistance. In central venous catheter-related infections due to coagulase-negative staphylococci, rifampin is sometimes added to vancomycin or oxacillin to facilitate eradication of the bacteria.

21. **C. Patients with pneumonic plague resulting from infection with *Y. pestis* appear ill with high fevers, productive coughs often with hemoptysis, and have chest x-ray findings showing multilobar involvement. Infected patients often have rapid clinical deterioration.**

Human metapneumovirus most commonly causes mild upper respiratory symptoms. In younger children, lower respiratory tract involvement leads to a bronchiolitis syndrome. This virus is most prevalent during the winter and early spring. Some centers can detect this virus by PCR testing of nasal aspirates.

BK virus usually causes infections in immunocompromised hosts, especially solid organ transplant recipients. Potential manifestations include viuria and hemorrhagic cystitis. Cidofovir may benefit some patients.

Smallpox presents early as a febrile syndrome with headache, myalgias, rigors, and vomiting. Following an incubation period of 7–17 days, ulcerative oral lesions appear, followed by a diffuse rash that develops into pustules, all in the same stage of healing throughout the body. There is no primary pulmonary symptom with smallpox infection.

22. **B. The MMR vaccination contain live attenuated viruses. Adults should receive a second dose of the MMR vaccination if they were previously vaccinated with a killed virus vaccine.**

    Precisely because of their immunocompromise, patients with HIV should receive pneumococcal polysaccharide vaccine boosters.

    The influenza inactivated virus vaccine is indicated only for pregnant women in their second and third trimesters during the influenza season.

    Hepatitis A vaccination is indicated for medical conditions (bleeding disorders requiring clotting factor concentrates, chronic liver disease), occupational exposures (people working with HAV in research settings), behavioral characteristics (illicit drug use, men who have sex with men), and for travel to areas of high/intermediate HAV prevalence. It is not routinely recommended for all health-care workers.

    Adults with a high-risk injury do not require a Td toxoid vaccination booster as long as the last vaccination was within 5 years.

23. **A. The combination of AZT/3TC (Combivir) with a protease inhibitor or nonnucleoside reverse transcriptase inhibitor has been established as a potent regimen with relatively few side effects.**

    AZT and D4T when combined exhibit intracellular antagonism.

    3TC and FTC differ only slightly in structure (5-fluoro substitution in FTC), and thus are considered similar drugs that should not be combined.

    D4T and DDI are known to have a marked increase in risk of fatal lactic acidosis, particularly in pregnancy.

    Triple NRTI regimens have been found to result in virologic failure and are not felt to be as potent as NRTI- or protease inhibitor-based regimens, and are not recommended as initial therapy.

24. **D. This patient has a localized skin and soft tissue infection for which oral outpatient therapy is indicated. His abscess was appropriately drained, with the Gram stain findings of gram-positive cocci in clusters being consistent with a staphylococcal infection. In addition, this patient is at high risk for methicillin-resistant *S. aureus* (MRSA) due to his use of injection drugs. MRSA isolates express an alternative penicillin-binding protein (PBP2a) with decreased affinity for beta-lactams. This leads to resistance to all beta-lactam antimicrobials (i.e., penicillins, cephalosporins, and carbapenems). TMP/SMX has very good empiric activity against MRSA with susceptibility rates of over 90% in most areas.**

    Most *S. aureus* produce a beta-lactamase that cleaves penicillin rendering it ineffective even for methicillin-susceptible *S. aureus* (MSSA).

    First generation cephalosporins are active against MSSA, but given the patient's risk factor for MRSA, cephalexin would not be an appropriate empiric choice.

The beta-lactamase inhibitor clavulanic acid would allow this antimicrobial combination to have activity against beta-lactamase-producing MSSA, but not MRSA, because PBP2a will still have low affinity for the amoxicillin.

Although there is geographic variation, the empiric susceptibilities of the fluoroquinolones are much less than that of TMP/SMX, roughly around 20% to 50%. In addition, because of concerns for the emergence of fluoroquinolone resistance, an alternative agent would be preferred when possible.

25. **B. Penicillin and other beta-lactam antimicrobials inhibit cell wall synthesis by binding to PBPs and preventing peptidoglycan cross-linking. Rates of penicillin-resistant *S. pneumoniae* have been increasing, with a national survey in 1999–2000 revealing 35% non-penicillin susceptibility (13% intermediate, 22% resistant). Penicillin-resistant *S. pneumoniae* expresses an altered PBP with decreased affinity for penicillin.**

    Efflux is a common mechanism of resistance for tetracyclines and is the most common mechanism in macrolide-resistant *S. pyogenes* in the US.

    Mutations in porin proteins, which function as channels through the outer bacterial cell membrane in gram-negative organisms, are an important example of decreased permeability leading to reduced antimicrobial susceptibility; however, this does not account for penicillin resistance in *S. pneumoniae*.

    Alteration of the ribosomal target would affect drugs targeting the ribosomes such as aminoglycosides, clindamycin, linezolid, macrolides, and streptogramins.

    S. pneumoniae does not express beta-lactamase enzymes. Beta-lactamases are frequently produced by *S. aureus*, as well as many of the gram-negative bacteria.

These doses are commonly prescribed but may vary by indication. Renal and hepatic disease may also affect recommended dosing. Please check an alternative source such as the Physicians' Desk Reference to confirm dosing and view information on side effects, drug interactions, and contraindications.

Acyclovir	Initial episode genital HSV: 200 mg 5 times per day
Amoxicillin	500–875 mg PO BID
Amoxicillin/clavulanate	500–875 mg PO BID
Azithromycin	Cervicitis due to *Chlamydia trachomatis*: 1 g PO once
	Mycobacterium avium complex prophylaxis for HIV-infected patients: 1200 mg PO each week
Cephalexin	250–500 mg PO BID–QID
Ciprofloxacin	500–750 mg PO BID
Fluconazole	100–800 mg PO QD depending on indication
	Bone marrow transplant fungal prophylaxis: 400 mg PO QD
	Vaginal candidiasis 150 mg PO once
Levofloxacin	500 mg PO BID
Linezolid	600 mg PO BID
Metronidazole	Giardiasis 250 mg PO TID
	Clostridium difficile colitis 250–500 mg PO QID
Moxifloxacin	400 mg PO QD
Trimethoprim-sulfamethoxazole	PCP prophylaxis: 1 DS tablet PO QD
	Alternative regimens: 1 DS tablet PO 3 times a week, or 1 SS tablet PO QD
	Higher doses used for treatment
Valacyclovir	Initial episode genital HSV: 1 g PO BID
	Recurrent episode genital HSV: 500 mg PO BID
	Herpes zoster: 1 g PO TID

Abbreviations: BID, twice daily; DS, double strength; HSV, herpes simplex virus; PCP, *Pneumocystis jiroveci* pneumonia; PO, oral; QD, daily; QID, four times daily; SS, single strength; TID, three times daily

Clinical Syndrome	Organisms	Primary Testing	Secondary Testing
Ophthalmologic Infections			
Keratitis/conjunctivitis			
Bacterial	*S. pneumoniae, H. influenzae, N. gonorrhoeae, Staphylococcus* spp, *Streptococcus* spp, GNR	DEC of corneal scrapings and/or exudate	
Viral	Adenovirus, HSV	Culture, antigen detection of corneal scrapings	
Fungal	*Aspergillus* spp, *Candida* spp, *Fusarium* spp	DEC of corneal scrapings	Fungal serology
Parasitic	*Acanthamoeba* spp, *Loa loa, Onchocerca volvulus, Toxocara canis*	DEC of corneal scrapings	Serology
Endophthalmitis/retinitis			
Bacterial	*Staphylococcus* spp, *P. aeruginosa, Bacillus* spp	DEC of intraocular aspirate	
Viral	HSV, CMV, VZV	Viral culture and antigen detection of intraocular aspirate	Serology
Fungal	*Candida* spp, *Aspergillus* spp, *H. capsulatum*	DEC of aspirate	Serology, urine antigen detection
Parasitic	*Toxoplasma gondii, Toxocara* spp, *Taenia solium, O. volvulus*	DEC of intraocular aspirate	NAT of intraocular aspirate
Orbital and periorbital cellulites: see Cellulitis, below			
CNS Infections			
Meningitis			
Bacterial	*S. pneumoniae, N. meningitidis, H. influenzae, L. monocytogenes, Rickettsia* spp, *Borrelia burgdorferi, Treponema pallidum, M. tuberculosis*	CSF analysis,[a] DEC	BC, acid-fast DEC, urine antigen detection, NAT
Viral	Enteroviruses, HIV, arboviruses	CSF analysis, viral culture, and NAT	Serology

(Continued)

Clinical Syndrome	Organisms	Primary Testing	Secondary Testing
Fungal	*Cryptococcus neoformans, Coccidioides immitis, Histoplasma capsulatum*	DEC, fungal serology, antigen detection	India ink prep, urine antigen detection
Parasitic	*Naegleria fowleri, Angiostrongylus cantonensis, Strongyloides stercoralis*	CSF DEC	Serology
Encephalitis			
Bacterial	*L. monocytogenes, T. pallidum, Actinomyces* spp, *Nocardia* spp, *M. tuberculosis*	CSF analysis, DEC; urine and blood antigen detection, serology	Brain biopsy, DEC
Viral	HSV, flaviviruses, rabies, HIV, enteroviruses	CSF analysis, viral culture, and NAT; serology	Viral culture and antigen detection of brain biopsy
Fungal	*C. neoformans, H. capsulatum*	CSF analysis, DEC, fungal serology, antigen detection	DEC and NAT of brain biopsy
Parasitic	*T. gondii, N. fowleri, Acanthamoeba*	DEC of biopsy specimen, serology	
Brain abscess			
Bacterial	*Streptococcus* spp (esp. *milleri* group), *S. aureus*, anaerobes, GNR	DEC of biopsy material, blood culture	
Fungal	*Candida* spp, *Aspergillus* spp, *Rhizopus* spp, *Pseudallescheria boydii, C. immitis, C. neoformans*	DEC of biopsy material	Antigen detection
Parasitic	*Trypanosoma cruzi, Entamoeba histolytica, Taenia solium, T. gondii, Schistosoma* spp, *Paragonimus* spp	DEC and antigen detection of biopsy specimen, serology	
Ventricular shunt infections			
Bacterial	*Staphylococcus* spp, *P. aeruginosa*, GNR, *Corynebacterium* spp	CSF DEC	
Ear, Nose, and Throat Infections			
Otitis externa			
Bacterial	*P. aeruginosa, S. aureus, S. pyogenes,*	DEC	
Fungal	*Aspergillus* spp, *Candida albicans*	DEC	
Otitis media			
Bacterial	*S. pneumoniae, H. influenzae, M. catarrhalis*	DEC of needle aspirate[b]	

Clinical Syndrome	Organisms	Primary Testing	Secondary Testing
Viral	Respiratory viruses	Viral culture, antigen detection	
Sinusitis			
Bacterial	*H. influenzae, S. pneumoniae, Staphylococcus* spp, *M. catarrhalis*, anaerobes	DEC of sinus aspirate[b]	
Viral	Respiratory viruses	Antigen detection, viral culture	
Fungal	*Aspergillus* spp, Zygomycetes	DEC of sinus aspirate	
Pharyngitis			
Bacterial	Group A *Streptococcus* (also group C), *C. diphtheriae, N. gonorrhoeae, C. pneumoniae, T. pallidum*	Rapid streptococcal antigen test, throat culture	Serology
Viral	Respiratory viruses, HSV, enteroviruses	Viral culture and antigen detection	Viral serologies
Laryngitis			
Bacterial	*M. catarrhalis, H. influenzae, M. tuberculosis*, beta-hemolytic Streptococci, *C. pneumoniae, M. pneumoniae*	Throat culture	Serology
Viral	Respiratory viruses	Viral culture, antigen detection	Serology
Fungal	*C. immitis, C. neoformans, H. capsulatum*	Fungal throat culture	Urine antigen detection
Respiratory Tract Infections			
Acute bronchitis			
Bacterial	*S. pneumoniae, H. influenzae, Bordetella pertussis, M. pneumoniae, C. pneumoniae, M. catarrhalis*	DEC, acute, and convalescent serologies	Special culture, PCR and/or antigen detection for *B. pertussis*
Viral	Respiratory viruses	Viral culture, antigen detection	
Community-acquired pneumonia			
Bacterial	Common: *S. pneumoniae, H. influenzae, S. aureus, M. pneumoniae, M. tuberculosis, C. pneumoniae*, anaerobes	DEC of sputum or BAL, acid-fast stain and culture, serology	BC, urine antigen detection, pleural biopsy and histopathology
	Less common: *Legionella, Chlamydia psittaci, Coxiella burnetii, Nocardia*	Require specialized media and/or growth conditions	NAT, serology, urine antigen detection

(*Continued*)

Clinical Syndrome	Organisms	Primary Testing	Secondary Testing
Viral	Respiratory viruses, SARS, hantavirus	Viral culture, antigen detection, serology	NAT
Fungal	*Aspergillus* spp, *H. capsulatum*, *C. immitis, Pneumocystis jiroveci*	DEC of sputum or BAL, antigen detection	Fungal NAT
Parasitic	*Ascaris lumbricoides, Strongyloides stercoralis, T. gondii, Paragonimus westermani*	Serology, antigen detection in BAL or biopsy	
Nosocomial pneumonia			
Bacterial	*P. aeruginosa, S. aureus*, GNR	DEC & sensitivities of sputum or BAL	
Viral	Respiratory viruses	Viral culture, antigen detection	
Empyema			
Bacterial	*Streptococcus* spp, *H. influenzae, M. tuberculosis, S. aureus*, GNR	Pleural fluid analysis, DEC, acid-fast stain and culture	BC, NAT of pleural fluid
Fungal	*H. capsulatum, C. immitis*	Pleural fluid analysis, DEC	Urine and blood antigen detection, serology
Parasitic	*E. histolytica*	Analysis, DEC of pleural fluid, antigen detection	Serology, antigen detection
Cardiac Infections			
Endocarditis			
Bacterial	Common: *Staphylococcus* spp, *Streptococcus* spp, *Enterococcus* spp, HACEK organisms, GNR	Three BCs at 1-hour intervals **before antibiotic therapy**	
	Less common: *Bartonella* spp, *C. burnetii, Chlamydia* spp, *Brucella* spp	Specialized culture, serology	
Fungal	*Candida* spp, *Aspergillus* spp	Three BCs at 1-hour intervals **before antibiotic therapy**	Antigen detection (blood)
Myocarditis			
Bacterial	*Corynebacterium diphtheriae, Clostridium perfringens*, group A *Streptococcus, Rickettsia* spp, *Legionella* spp, *B. burgdorferi, M. pneumoniae*	BC, serology	DEC of endomyocardial biopsy, urine antigen detection

Clinical Syndrome	Organisms	Primary Testing	Secondary Testing
Viral	Enteroviruses, respiratory viruses, measles, arboviruses	Viral culture and serology	Heart biopsy
Fungal	*Aspergillus* spp, *Candida* spp, *Cryptococcus* spp	Fungal serology	DEC of endomyocardial biopsy
Parasitic	*Trypanosoma* spp, *Trichinella spiralis*, *T. gondii*	Thick & thin blood smear, serology	Examination of endomyocardial biopsy
Pericarditis			
Bacterial	*S. pneumoniae*, *S. aureus*, *Neisseria* spp, *Mycoplasma* spp, *Mycobacterium* spp	BC, DEC of pericardial fluid, AFB stain and culture	Urine antigen detection
Viral	Enteroviruses, adenovirus, HSV	Culture of pericardial fluid, serology, antigen detection	
Fungal	*H. capsulatum*, *Blastomyces dermatitidis*, *C. immitis*, *C. neoformans*, *Aspergillus* spp, *Candida* spp	DEC of pericardial fluid, serology, antigen detection	Urine antigen detection
Parasitic	*T. gondii*, *E. histolytica*, *T. canis*, *Schistosoma* spp	Serology, direct exam of pericardial fluid, antigen detection	
Gastrointestinal Tract Infections			
Gastroenteritis			
Bacterial	*Salmonella* spp, *Shigella* spp, *E. coli*, *Campylobacter* spp, *Vibrio* spp, *Yersinia* spp	Stool culture	
Viral	Rotavirus, norovirus, adenovirus	Culture, antigen detection	
Parasitic	*Giardia lamblia*, *E. histolytica*, *Balantidium coli*, *Microsporidium* spp, *Cryptosporidium parvum*, *Cyclospora cayetanensis*, *Isospora belli*	O&P exam, antigen detection, AFB stain	Serology
Antibiotic-associated colitis			
Bacterial	*Clostridium difficile*	EIA, culture and toxin testing, NAT	

(Continued)

Clinical Syndrome	Organisms	Primary Testing	Secondary Testing
Hepatitis			
Viral	Hepatitis A through E	Serology	
Peptic ulcer disease			
Bacterial	*Helicobacter pylori*	Stool antigen detection, urea breath test, serology	Culture
Genitourinary Tract Infections			
Urinary tract infections			
Bacterial	*E. coli, Staphylococcus* spp, GNR	Urinalysis, Gram stain	Culture
Fungal	*Candida* spp	DEC	
Parasitic	*Schistosoma haematobium*	Exam for eggs in urine sediment	Stool O&P, rectal biopsy, serology
Genital skin and mucosal lesions			
Bacterial	*T. pallidum, N. gonorrhoeae, Haemophilus ducreyi*	VDRL, RPR; DEC including darkfield microscopy of lesion	NAT
Viral	HSV	Antigen detection, culture	NAT
Cervicitis			
Bacterial	*Chlamydia trachomatis, N. gonorrhoeae,* actinomycetes, *T. pallidum*	DEC, NAT, serology	
Viral	HSV, HPV, adenovirus	Viral culture, antigen detection	Serology
Parasitic	*Trichomonas vaginalis*	Direct exam	Culture
Vulvovaginitis			
Bacterial	*Gardnerella vaginalis,* anaerobes, *M. hominis, Ureaplasma urealyticum*	Direct exam	
Fungal	*C. albicans,* other *Candida* spp	DEC	
Parasitic	*T. vaginalis*	DEC	
Urethritis			
Bacterial	*N. gonorrhoeae, C. trachomatis, U. urealyticum, M. genitalium*	DEC, antigen detection, NAT	
Viral	HSV	Culture, antigen detection	
Parasitic	*Trichomonas* spp	Wet mount direct exam	Culture

Clinical Syndrome	Organisms	Primary Testing	Secondary Testing
Skin and Soft Tissue Infections			
Infections following bites			
Bacterial	*Capnocytophaga canimorsus, Pasteurella* spp, oral anaerobes, *Staphylococcus* spp, *Streptococcus* spp, *Eikenella corrodens*	DEC	
Cellulitis			
Bacterial	*S. aureus, Streptococcus* spp., *Erysipelothrix rhusiopathiae, Mycobacterium* spp, GNR	DEC of needle aspirate or biopsy material	BC
Vesicular lesions			
Viral	VZV, HSV, poxviruses	Viral culture and antigen detection	Serology
Ulcerative lesions			
Bacterial	*Mycobacterium* spp, *Bacillus anthracis, Francisella tularensis, T. pallidum, C. diphtheriae*	DEC of lesion	Serology
Parasitic	*Leishmania* spp	DEC of lesion	NAT, blood smears
Necrotizing fasciitis			
Bacterial	*S. pyogenes, S. aureus, C. perfringens,* anaerobes, GNR	DEC of biopsy material, BC	
Bone and Joint Infections			
Infectious arthritis			
Bacterial	*N. gonorrhoeae, S. aureus, H. influenzae, M. tuberculosis,* beta-hemolytic Streptococci, GNR, *C. trachomatis*	Analysis of joint fluid, DEC	BC
Fungal	*Sporothrix schenckii, C. immitis, B. dermatitidis, Candida* spp	Analysis of joint fluid, DEC	BC
Viral	Rubella, hepatitis B, parvovirus B-19	Viral serology	NAT
Osteomyelitis			
Bacterial	*S. aureus, Streptococcus* spp, GNR, anaerobes	BC, DEC of biopsy specimen	
Fungal	*Candida* spp, *C. neoformans, B. dermatitidis, C. immitis*	BC, DEC of biopsy specimen	Serology, antigen detection

(*Continued*)

Clinical Syndrome	Organisms	Primary Testing	Secondary Testing
Bloodstream Infections			
Sepsis			
Bacterial	GNR, *Staphylococcus* spp, *Streptococcus* spp	BC	
Fungal	*Candida* spp	BC	
Central venous catheter-related infections			
Bacterial	*Staphylococcus* spp, *Streptococcus* spp, *Pseudomonas* spp, GNR	Paired BC drawn through CVC and peripheral site	Quantitative BCs of line and peripheral site, culture catheter tip
Fungal	*Candida* spp	Paired BC drawn through CVC and peripheral site	Quantitative BCs of line and peripheral site, culture catheter tip
Toxic shock syndrome			
Bacterial	*S. aureus, S. pyogenes*	DEC of infected site, BC	
Miscellaneous			
Parasitic	*Plasmodium* spp, *Babesia microti, T. cruzi, Leishmania* spp	Thick and thin blood smear, serology	NAT

[a] Fluid analysis should include cell count with differential, glucose, protein
[b] Cultures of respiratory flora and/or nasal secretions are not useful for diagnosis of bacterial sinusitis or otitis media

Abbreviations: AFB, acid-fast bacilli; BAL, bronchoalveolar lavage; BC, blood culture; CMV, cytomegalovirus; CSF, cerebrospinal fluid; CVC, central venous catheter; DEC, direct examination and culture; GNR, gram-negative rods; HSV, herpes simplex virus; NAT, nucleic acid testing (including PCR, RT-PCR, LCR, FISH, molecular probes, etc.); SARS; sudden acute respiratory syndrome; VZV, varicella-zoster virus

Evidence-Based Resources

CHAPTER 3

Appelbaum PC. Resistance among *Streptococcus pneumoniae*: Implications for drug selection. Clin Infect Dis 2002;34: 1613–1620.

Chang S, Sievert DM, Hageman JC, et al. Infection with vancomycin-resistant *Staphylococcus aureus* containing the *vanA* resistance gene. N Engl J Med 2003;348:1342–1347.

Davidson R, Cavalcanti R, Brunton JL, et al. Resistance to levofloxacin and failure of treatment of pneumococcal pneumonia. N Engl J Med 2002;346:747–750.

Murray BE. Vancomycin-resistant enterococcal infections. N Engl J Med 2000;342:710–721.

Naimi TS, LeDell KH, Como-Sabetti K, et al. Comparison of community- and health care-associated methicillin-resistant *Staphylococcus aureus* infection. JAMA 2003;290:2976–2984.

Scheld WM. Maintaining fluoroquinolone class efficacy: Review of influencing factors. Emerg Infect Dis 2003;9:1–9.

CHAPTER 5

Balfour HH. Drug therapy: Antiviral drugs. N Engl J Med 1999; 340:1255–1268.

Guidelines for the Use of Antiretroviral Agents in HIV-1-Infected Adults and Adolescents (DHHS). Web site. Available at: http://www.aidsinfo.nih.gov. Accessed March 23, 2004.

Jefferson T, Demicheli V, Deeks J, Rivetti D. Neuraminidase inhibitors for preventing and treating influenza in healthy adults. Cochrane Database Syst Rev. 2000;(2):CD001265. Review.

CHAPTER 6

Brodovsky SC, Snibson GR. Corneal and conjunctival infections. Curr Opin Ophthalmol 1997;8:2–7.

Herpetic Eye Disease Study Group (HEDS). Oral acyclovir for HSV eye disease: Effect on prevention of epithelial keratitis and stromal keratitis. Arch Ophthalmol 2000;118:1030–1036.

Van Bijsterveld OP, Jager GV. Infectious diseases of the conjunctiva and cornea. Curr Opin Ophthalmol 1996;7:65–70.

CHAPTER 7

Durand MI, Calderwood SB, Weber DJ, et al. Acute bacterial meningitis in adults. New Engl J Med 1993;328:21–28.

Gans JD, Beek DVD. Dexamethasone in adults with bacterial meningitis. N Engl J Med 2002;347:1549–1556.

Hasbun R, Abrahms J, Jekel J, Quagliarello VJ. Computed tomography of the head before lumbar puncture in adults with suspected meningitis. N Engl J Med 2001;345:1727–1733.

Johnson RT. Acute encephalitis. Clin Infect Dis 1996;23:219–226.

Pruitt AA. Infections of the nervous system. Neurol Clin 1998; 16:419–447.

Spanos A, Harrell FE, Durack DT. Differential diagnosis of acute meningitis. JAMA 1989;262:2700–2707.

CHAPTER 8

Anon JB, Jacobs MR, Poole MD, et al. Antimicrobial treatment guidelines for acute bacterial rhinosinusitis. Otolaryngol Head Neck Surg 2004;130:1–45.

Benninger MS, Ferguson BJ, Hadley JA, et al. Adult chronic rhinosinusitis: definitions, diagnosis, epidemiology, and pathophysiology. Otolaryngol Head Neck Surg 2003;129:S1–S32.

Bisno AL, et al. Diagnosis and management of group A streptococcal pharyngitis: A practice guideline. Infectious Diseases Society of America. Clin Infect Dis 1997;25:574–583.

Fairbanks DN. Pocket Guide to Antimicrobial Therapy in Otolaryngology—Head and Neck Surgery. 10th ed. Alexandria: American Academy of Otolaryngology, Head and Neck Surgery Foundation, 2001.

Manolidis S, et al. Comparative efficacy of aminoglycoside versus fluoroquinolone topical antibiotic drops. Otolaryngol Head Neck Surg 2004;130:S83–S88.

Vincent MT, Celestin N, Hussain AN. Pharyngitis. Am Fam Physician 2004;69:1465–1470.

CHAPTER 9

American Thoracic Society, CDC, Infectious Diseases Society of America. Treatment of tuberculosis. MMWR Recomm Rep 2003;52:1–77.

Joseph J, Barinath P, Bascan GS, Sahn SA. Is the pleural fluid transudate or exudate? A revisit of the diagnostic criteria. Thorax 2001;56:867–870.

Mandell LA, Bartlett JG, Dowell SF, et al. Update of practice guidelines for the management of community-acquired pneumonia in immunocompetent adults. Clin Infect Dis 2003;37: 1405–1433. Epub 2003 Nov 03.

Niederman MS, Mandell LA, Anzueto A, et al. Guidelines for the management of adults with community-acquired pneumonia. Diagnosis, assessment of severity, antimicrobial therapy, and prevention. Am J Respir Crit Care Med 2001;163:1730–1754.

CHAPTER 10

Feldman AM, McNamara D. Myocarditis. N Engl J Med 2000; 343:1388–1398.

Moreillon P, Que Y. Infective endocarditis. Lancet 2004;363: 139–149.

Troughton RW, Asher CR, Klein AL. Pericarditis. Lancet 2004;363: 717–727.

CHAPTER 11

DuPont HL. Guidelines on acute infectious diarrhea in adults. Am J Gastroenterol 1997;92:1962–1975.

EASL International Consensus Conference on Hepatitis B. J Hepatol 2003;39:S3–S25.

Harris JC, DuPont HL, Hornick RB. Fecal leukocytes in diarrheal illness. Ann Int Med 1972;76:697–703.

National Institutes of Health consensus development conference statement: management of hepatitis C: 2002—June 10–12, 2002. Hepatology. 2002 Nov;36(5 Suppl 1):S3–20.

Yassin SF, Young-Fadok TM, Zein NN, Pardi DS. *Clostridium difficile*-associated diarrhea and colitis. Mayo Clin Proc 2001; 76:725–730.

CHAPTER 12

Kimberlin DW, Rouse DJ. Genital herpes. N Engl J Med 2004; 350:1970–1977.

Workowski KA, Levine, WC. Sexually transmitted diseases treatment guidelines—2002. Centers for Disease Control and Prevention. MMWR Recomm Rep 2002;51:1–78.

Web site. Available at: http://www.cdc.gov/STD/treatment. Accessed March 17, 2005.

CHAPTER 13

Green RJ, Dafoe DC, Raffin TA. Necrotizing fasciitis. Chest 1996;110:219–229.

Hirschmann JV. Impetigo: Diagnosis and management. In: Swartz M, Remington JS, eds. Current Clinical Topics in Infectious Diseases 22. Malden, MA: Blackwell Publishing, 2002:42–51.

Swarz MN. Clinical practice. Cellulitis. N Engl J Med 2004;26: 904–912.

Talan DA, Citron DM, Abrahamian FM, et al. Bacteriologic analysis of infected dog and cat bites. N Engl J Med 1999;340: 85–92.

CHAPTER 14

Goldenberg DL, Reed JI. Bacterial arthritis. N Engl J Med 1985;312:764–771.

Lew DP, Waldvogel FA. Osteomyelitis. Lancet 2004;364: 369–379.

Lew DP, Waldvogel FA. Osteomyelitis. N Engl J Med 1997; 336:999.

Mader JT, Shirtliff M, Calhoun JH. Staging and staging application in osteomyelitis. Clin Infect Dis 1997;25:1303.

Smith JW, Piercy EA. Infectious arthritis. Clin Infec Dis 1995;20:225–231.

Waldvogel FA, Medoff G, Swartz MN. Osteomyelitis: A review of clinical features, therapeutic considerations, and unusual aspects. N Engl J Med 1970; 282:198.

CHAPTER 15

Bernard GR, Vincent JL, Laterre PF, et al. Efficacy and safety of recombinant human activated protein C for severe sepsis. N Engl J Med 2001; 344:699–709.

Mermel LA, Farr BM, Sherertz RJ, et al. Guidelines for the management of intravascular catheter-related infections. Clin Infect Dis 2001;32:1249–1272.

Raad I, Hanna HA, Alakech B, et al. Differential time to positivity: a useful method for diagnosing catheter-related bloodstream infections. Ann Intern Med 2004;140:18–25.

CHAPTER 16

US Department of Health and Human Services. Post-exposure prophylaxis: Health-care worker guidelines. Web site. Available at: http://aidsinfo.nih.gov/guidelines.

US Department of Health and Human Services. Management of HIV complications: Prevention of opportunistic infections guidelines. Web site. Available at: http://aidsinfo.nih.gov/guidelines.

Yeni PG, Hammer SM, Hirsch MS, et al. Treatment for adult HIV infection: 2004 recommendations of the International AIDS Society—USA Panel. JAMA 2004;292(2):251–265.

CHAPTER 17

Bisharat N, Omari H, Raz R. Risk of infection and death among post-splenectomy patients. J Infect 2001;43:182–186.

Dykewicz CA. Summary of the guidelines for preventing opportunistic infections among hematopoietic stem cell transplant patients. Clin Infect Dis 2001;33:139–144.

Fishman JA, Rubin RH. Infection in organ-transplant recipients. N Engl J Med 1998;338:1741–1751.

Hughes WT, Armstrong D, Bodey GP, et al. 2002 Guidelines for the use of antimicrobial agents in neutropenic patients with cancer. Clin Infect Dis 2002;34:730–751.

Working Party of the British Committee for Standards in Haematology Clinical Haematology Task Force. Guidelines for the prevention and treatment of infection in patients with an absent or dysfunctional spleen. BMJ 1996;312:430–434.

CHAPTER 18

Drenth J, van der Meer J. Medical progress: Hereditary periodic fever. New Engl J Med 2001;345:1748–1757.

Grateau G. Clinical and genetic aspects of the hereditary periodic fever syndromes. Rheumatology 2004 Apr;43;410–415.

Knockaert DC, Dujardin KS, Bobbaers HJ. Long-term follow-up of patients with undiagnosed fever of unknown origin. Arch Intern Med 1996;156:618–620.

McGinley-Smith D, Tsao S. Dermatoses from ticks. J Am Acad Derm 2003;49:363–392.

Steere A, Cobum J, Glickstein L. The emergence of Lyme Disease. J Clin Invest 2004;113:1093–1101.

Vanderschueren S, Knockaert D, Adriaenssens T, Demey W, Durnez A, Blockmans D, Bobbaers H. From prolonged febrile illness to FUO. Arch Intern Med 2003;163:1033–1041.

Wormser GP, Nadelman RB, Dattwyler RJ, et al. Practice guidelines for the treatment of Lyme disease. The Infectious Diseases Society of America. Clin Infect Dis 2000;31:1–14.

CHAPTER 19

Humar, Keystone. Evaluating fever in travellers returning from tropical countries. Brit Med J 1996;312:953–956.

Kain KC. Skin lesions in returned travelers. Med Clin N Am 1999;83:1077–1102.

Ryan ET, Wilson ME, Kain KC. Illness after international travel. NEJM 2002;347:505–516.

Spira AM. Assessment of travellers who return home ill. Lancet 2003;361:1459–1469.

Spira AM. Preparing the traveller. Lancet 2003;361:1368–1381.

CHAPTER 20

Breman JG, Henderson DA. Diagnosis and management of smallpox. N Engl J Med 2002;346:1300–1308.

Centers for Disease Control and Prevention. Emergency preparedness and response. Web site. Available at: http://www.bt.cdc.gov. Accessed March 18, 2005.

Centers for Disease Control and Prevention. Recognition of illness associated with the intentional release of a biological agent. MMWR 2001;50:890–897.

Cherry CL, Kainer MA, Ruff TA. Biological weapons preparedness: the role of physicians. Intern Med J 2003;33:242–253.

Shafazand S. When bioterrorism strikes: diagnosis and management of inhalational anthrax. Semin Resp Infect 2003;18:134–145.

Index

Note: Page numbers with a *t* indicate tables; those with a *b* indicate boxes.